I0049953

The Bare Minimum: Donatelli Shoulder Method
Assessment and Treatment

2nd Edition

Donn Dimond, PT, OCS
Robert Donatelli, PT, PhD, OCS
Kent Morimatsu, DPT

**For more "The Bare Minimum" books check out our website: www.thebareminimum.net
or check out www.amazon.com
If you would like to contact the authors for questions please email us at
dimondpt@gmail.com.**

Copyright © 2011 by Donn Dimond

All rights reserved.
Published in the United States

Notice.

Physical Therapy is an ever changing field and standard safety precautions must be followed. As new research and clinical experience broaden our knowledge, changes in treatment may become necessary or appropriate. It is the responsibility of the treating physical therapist to determine the best treatment for each individual patient. Neither the publisher nor the author assume any liability for any injury and or damage to persons or property arising from this publication.

ISBN: 978-0-9821394-9-3

2nd Edition

CONTENTS

Mobility Tests

Shoulder Flexion

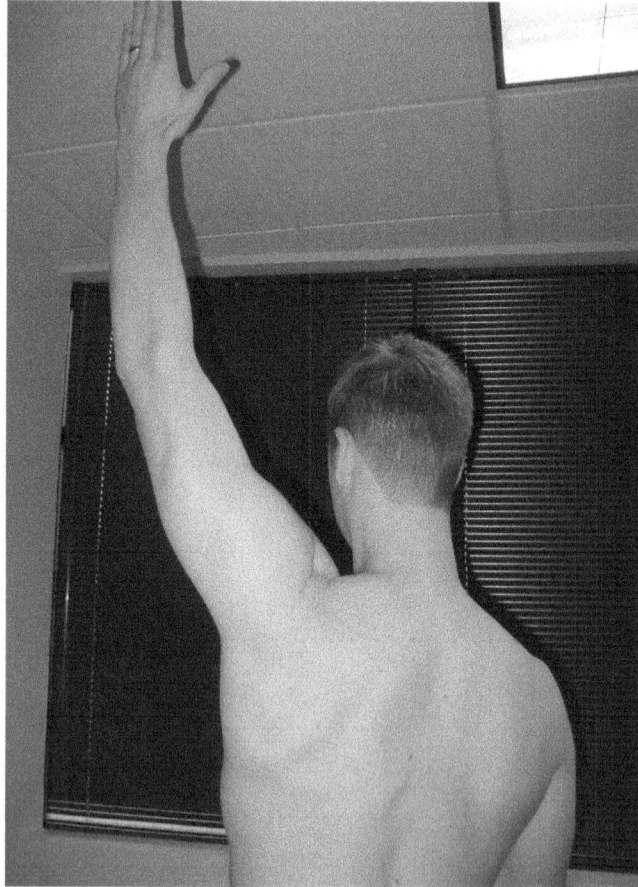

- With the patient standing, the patient raises their arm up as high as they can in the position of scaption (POS), 30-45 degrees anterior to frontal plane.
- The therapist also notes how well the humerus "disassociates" from the scapula in the last phase of elevation (140 to 180 degrees).

If the patient is restricted in this motion, think limitations in subscapularis, teres minor, or posterior capsule.

Shoulder ER at 0 deg Abduction

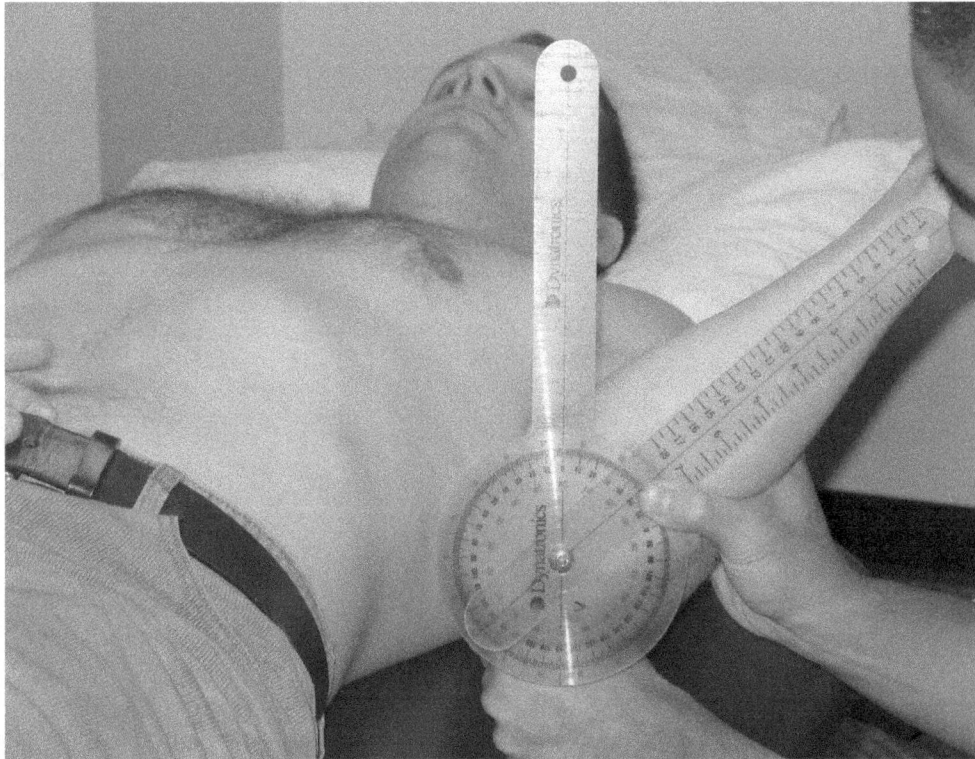

- While the patient is lying on their back, therapist holds the patient's arm with one hand in midline.
- The other hand holds a goniometer to the patient's forearm and rotates the forearm away from the patient's body until the therapist feels the slack being taken up. The PT measures the amount of rotation.

If the patient is restricted in this motion, think limitations in subscapularis muscle length or possible coracohumerall ligament restriction.

Treatment: Mobilize subscap first with techniques on page 36. If this doesn't work then mobilize coracoacrominal ligament with technique on pages 38-39

Shoulder ER at 90 abduction and position of scaption (around 30 deg anterior to frontal plane)

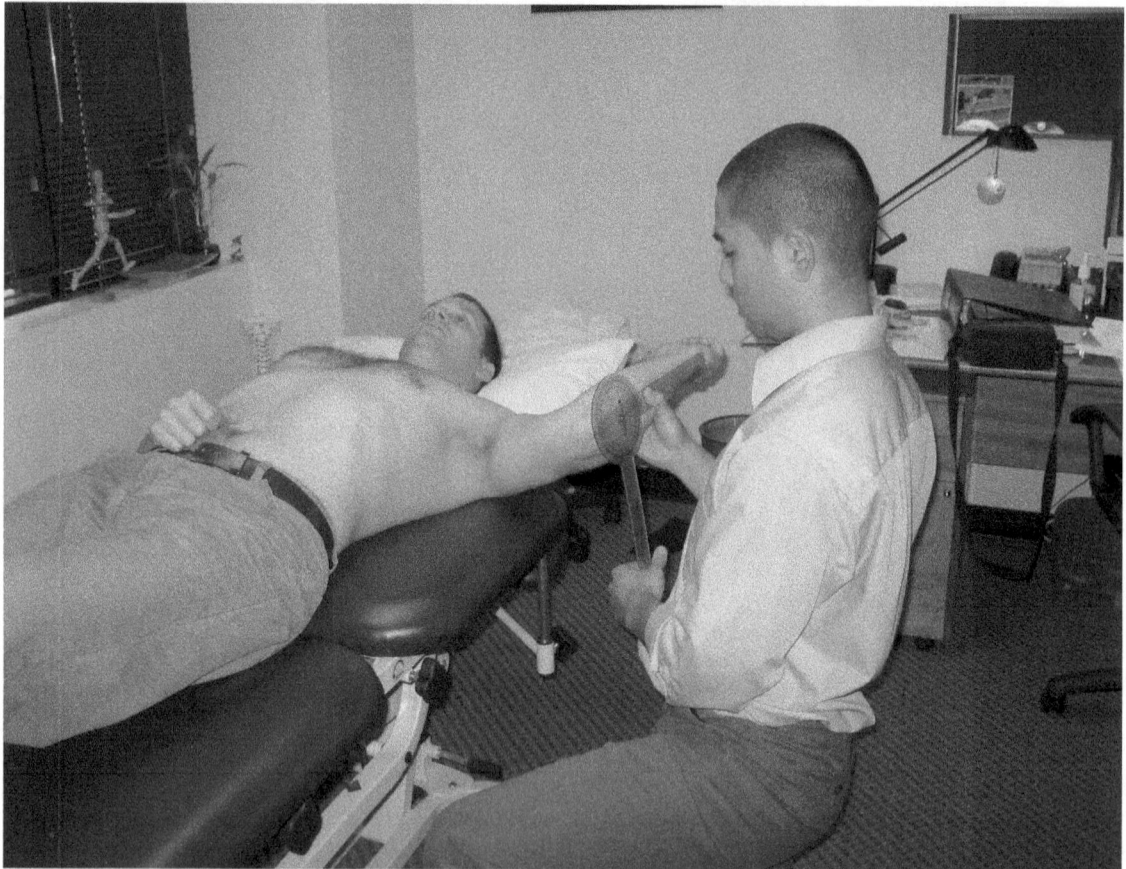

- With the patient in supine, the therapist moves the patient's arm into 90 degrees abduction.
- The therapist then externally rotates the patient's arm until the therapist feels that the slack has been taken up.

If the patient is restricted in this motion, think limitation in the Inferior Glenohumeral Ligament Complex (IGHL)

Treatment: Mobilize the IGHL with technique on page 40.

Internal Rotation in side lying

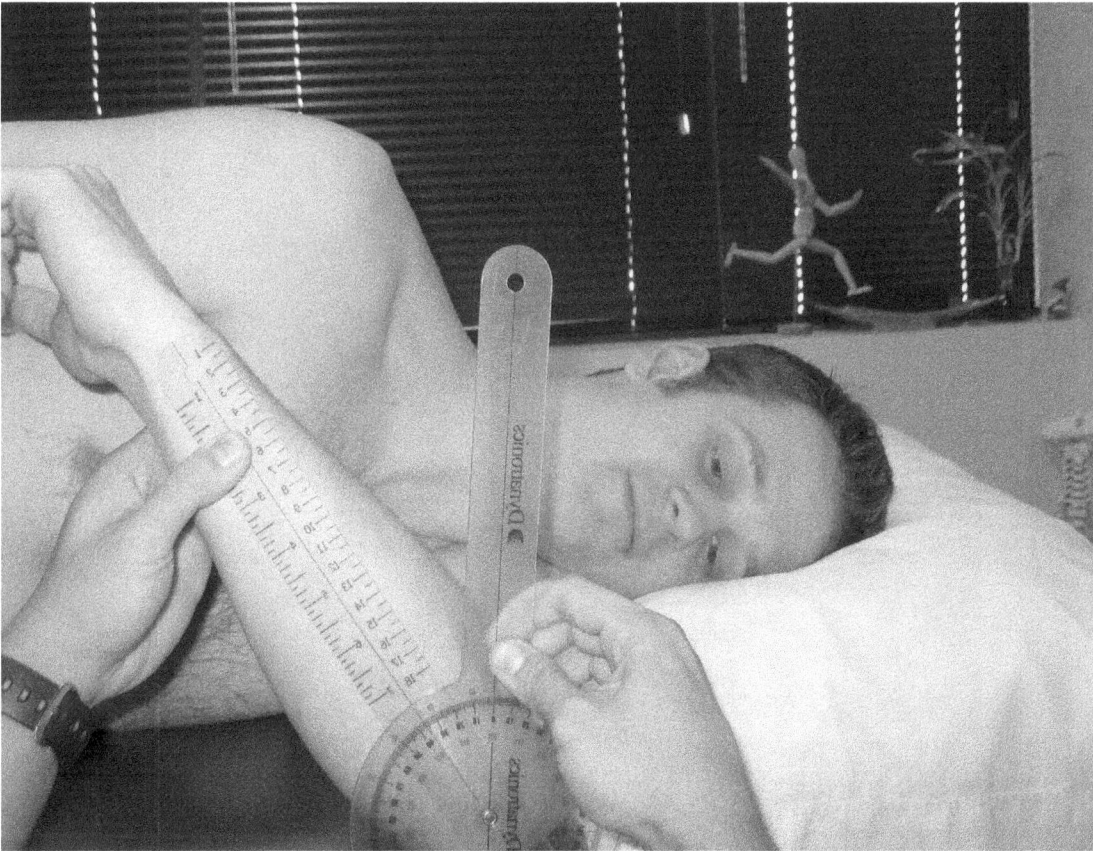

- With the patient in side lying, the arm is placed in 90 degrees of flexion in the sagittal plane with the elbow bent at 90 degrees.
- The therapist then rotates the patient's arm inferiorly towards the patient's hips until the slack is taken up in the patient's shoulder, being careful to make sure that the patient's shoulder doesn't start to rise off the table. The therapist then measures the angle of rotation.

If the patient is restricted in this motion, think limitation in the overall posterior capsule.

Treatment: Mobilize the posterior capsule with techniques from pages 41-43.

30E of extension & internal rotation

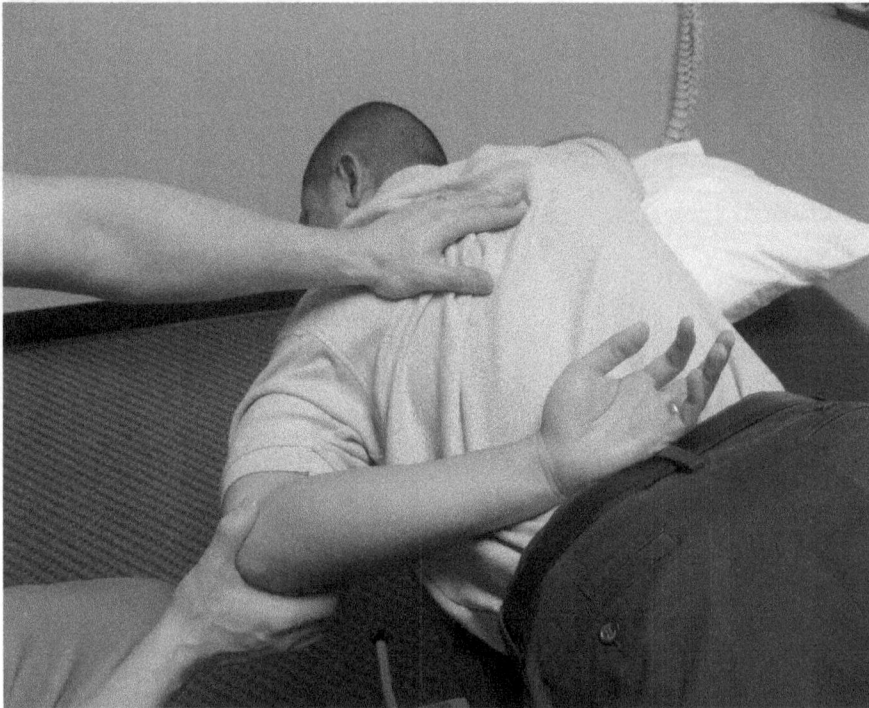

- While the patient is lying on their stomach, the therapist moves the patient's arm into 30 degrees of shoulder extension.
- While the hand is resting on the patient's waist the therapist pushes the patient's shoulder blade against their rib cage.
- The distance from the patient's elbow to the plinth can be noted and compared to the other arm.

If the patient is restricted in this motion, think limitation in the inferior fibers of the posterior capsule

Treatment: Mobilize the posterior capsule with techniques from page 43.

Internal rotation in 30E abduction in the Plane of Scapula

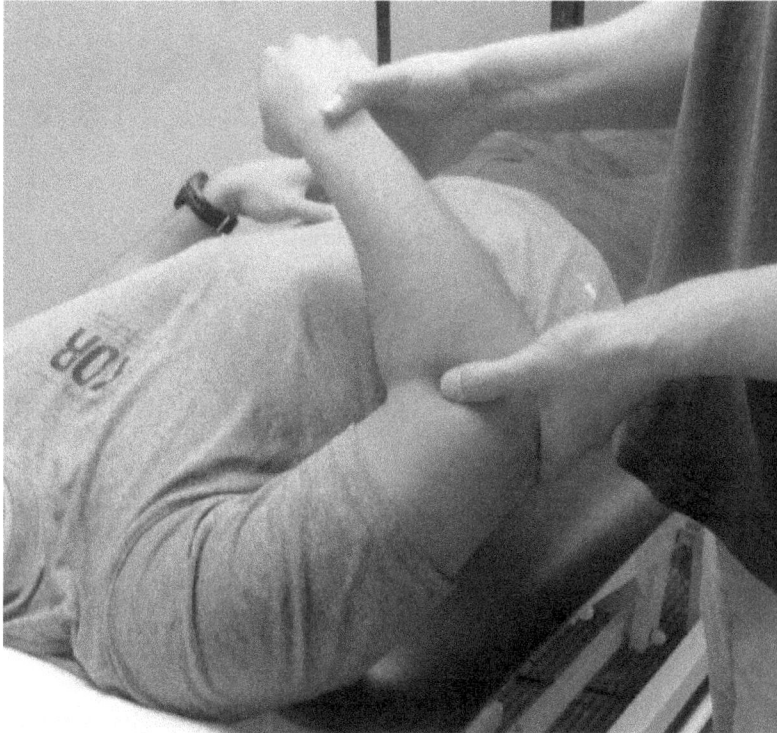

- With the patient lying on their back, the therapist moves the arm into 30degrees abduction while maintaining the position of scaption.
- The therapist then internally rotates the patient's arm down and takes a measurement with their goniometer.

If the patient is restricted in this motion, think limitation in the Superior and Middle fibers of posterior capsule

Treatment: Mobilize the posterior capsule with techniques from pages 41-42.

60E abduction in frontal plane & internal rotation

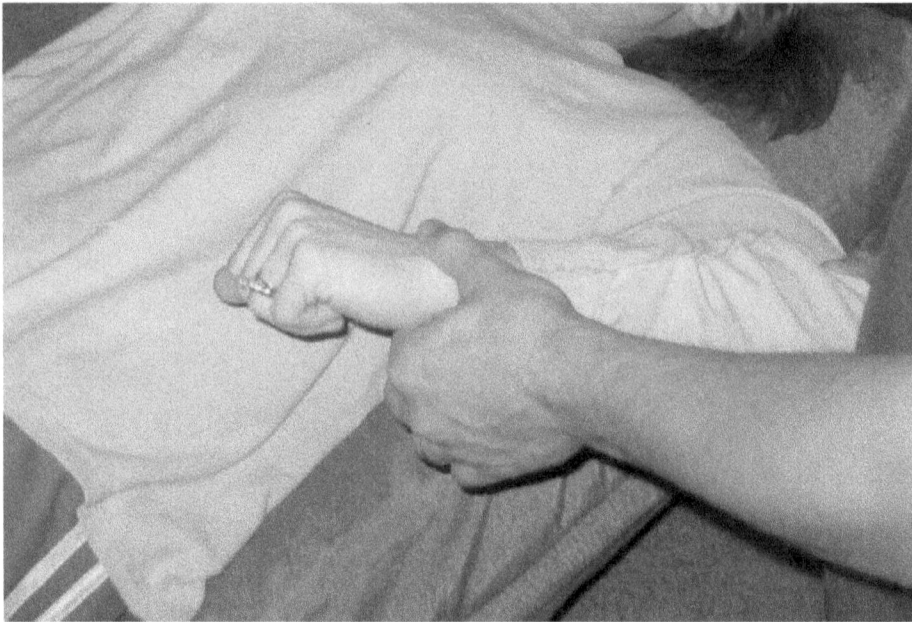

- With the patient lying on their back, the therapist brings the patient's out to 60 degrees abduction.
- The therapist then rotates the arm down until the slack is taken up while making sure not to allow the shoulder to come off the table. The therapist can then make a note of the ROM

If the patient is restricted in this motion, think limitation in the posterior capsule in general

Treatment: Mobilize the posterior capsule with techniques from pages 41-42.

Strength Tests

Infraspinatus

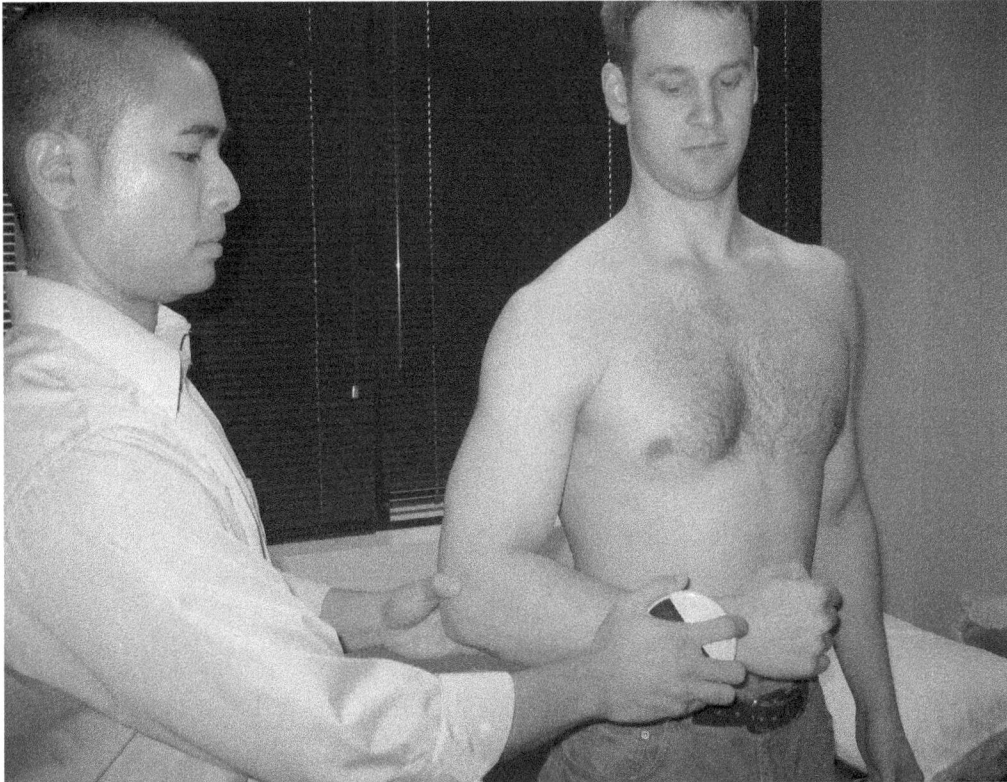

- The patient stands with the arm at the side with the elbow at 90° and the humerus medially rotated to 45°.
- The examiner then applies a medial rotation force that the patient resists. Counter pressure is applied by the examiner against the inner aspect of the distal end of the humerus in order to ensure a rotation movement.

Treatment: If weak, strengthen this muscle with the exercises on pages 52, 53,59,60,61, 66.

Kelly BT, Kadrmas WR, Speer KP. The manual muscle examination for rotator cuff strength: An electromyographic investigation. *Am. J. Sports Med.*, 24: 581–588, 1996.
Magee DJ. *Orthopedic Physical Assessment*. 4th ed. 2002, Philadelphia: Saunders

Supraspinatus

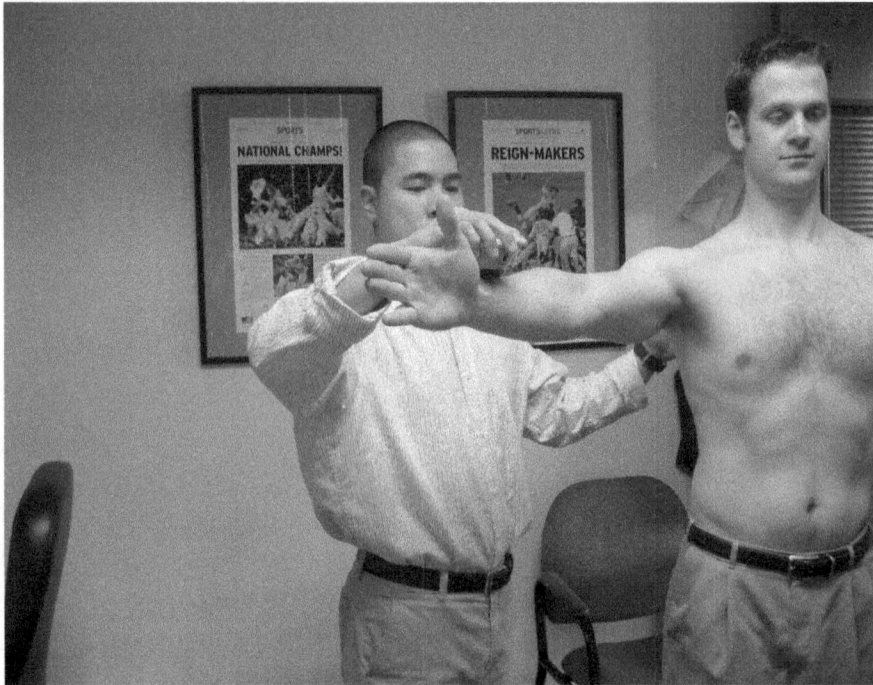

- The patient elevates the arm to 90° in the scapular plane in the "full can" position with the thumb pointing up.
- The patient is asked to resist as the examiner applies a downward force to the distal forearm. Kelly et. al, found no significant difference in suprapinatus muscle activation when comparing the "full can" and "empty can" positions.
- Furthermore, the "full can" activated the infraspinatus muscle significantly less and avoids the positional pain provocation associated with the "empty can" position.

<u>Treatment:</u> If weak, strengthen this muscle with the exercises on pages 50, 53, 59,60,61,66.

Kelly BT, Kadrmas WR, Speer KP. The manual muscle examination for rotator cuff strength: An electromyographic investigation. *Am. J. Sports Med.*, 24: 581–588, 1996.
Magee DJ. *Orthopedic Physical Assessment*. 4th ed. 2002, Philadelphia: Saunders

Subscapularis

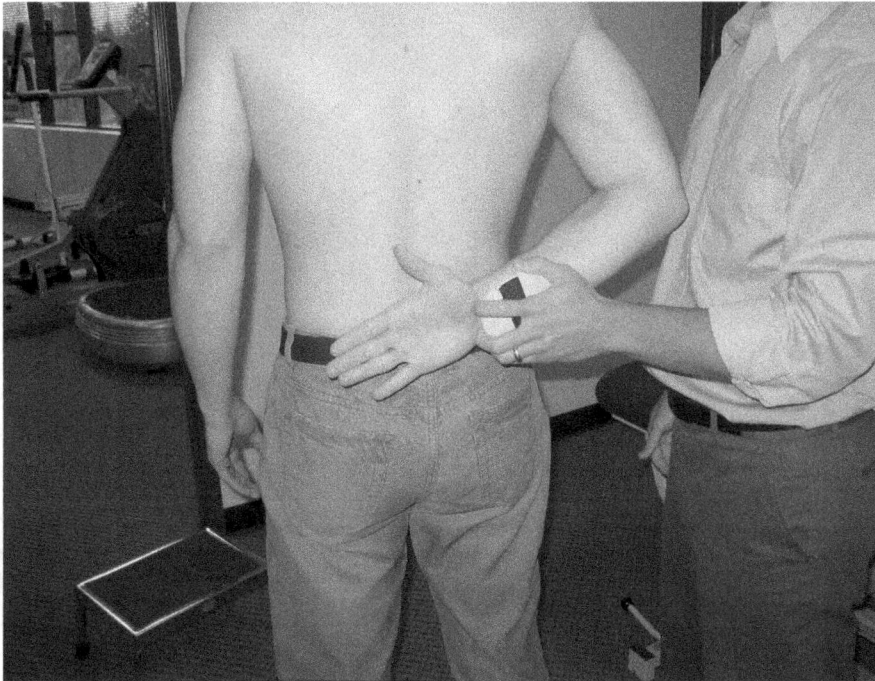

- The patient places the dorsum of the hand against the mid lumbar supine.
- The patient is instructed to take the hand away from the back and the examiner applies a load pushing the hand toward the back.
- This test maximizes subscapularis muscle activation and minimizes the activation from the pectoralis and latissimus muscles.

Treatment: If weak, strengthen this muscle with the exercises on pages 54,60,65,67.

Kelly BT, Kadrmas WR, Speer KP. The manual muscle examination for rotator cuff strength: An electromyographic investigation. *Am. J. Sports Med.*, 24: 581–588, 1996.
Gerber C, Hersche O, Farron A. Isolated rupture of the subscapularis tendon. *J Bone Joint Surg Am* 1996; 78:1015-23.
Greis PE, et al. Validation of the Lift-Off Test and Analysis of Subscapularis Activity During Maximal Internal Rotation. *Am. J. Sports Med.* 24: 589-593, 1996

Serratus Anterior

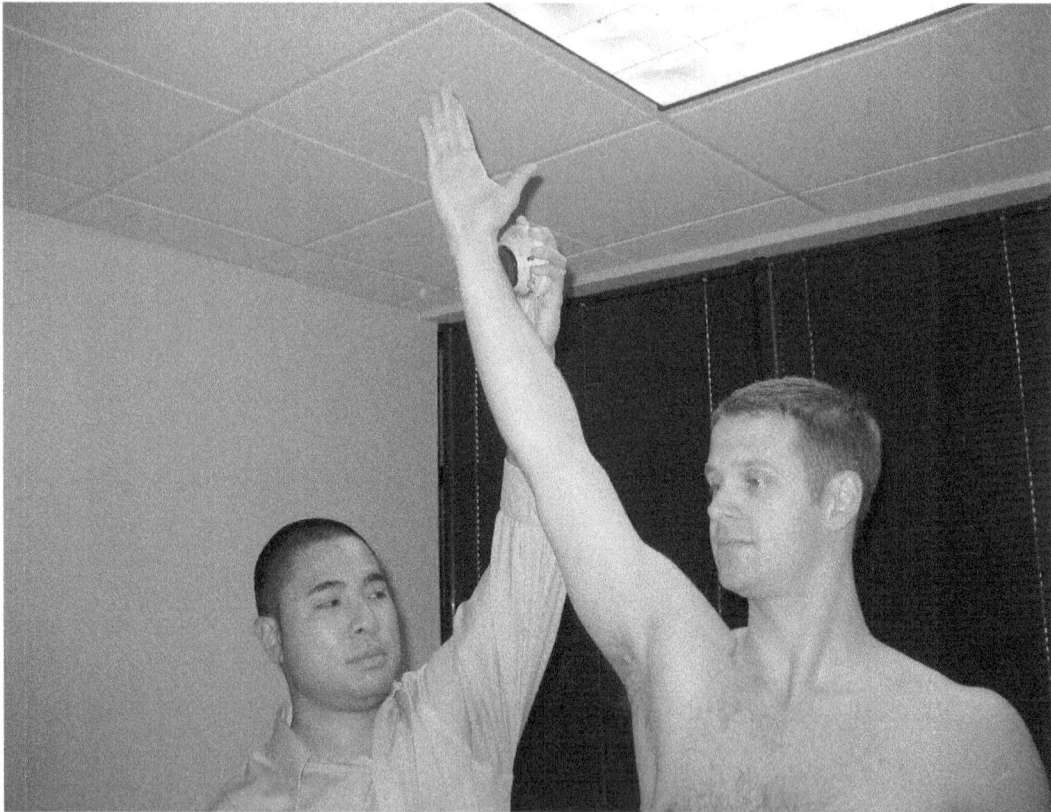

- The patient's arm is elevated to 125° in the scapular plane
- The patient is instructed to resist as the examiner applies downward pressure to the distal forearm.
- Ekstrom et. al demonstrated high serratus anterior EMG activity as the scapula upwardly rotates above 120° of shoulder elevation.

Treatment: If weak, strengthen this muscle with the exercises on pages 48,57,63,64.

Ekstrom RA, Donatelli RA, Soderberg GL. Surface electromyographic analysis of exercises for the trapezius and serratus anterior muscles. *J Orthop Sports Phys Ther*. 33:247-258, 2008.

Lower Trapezius

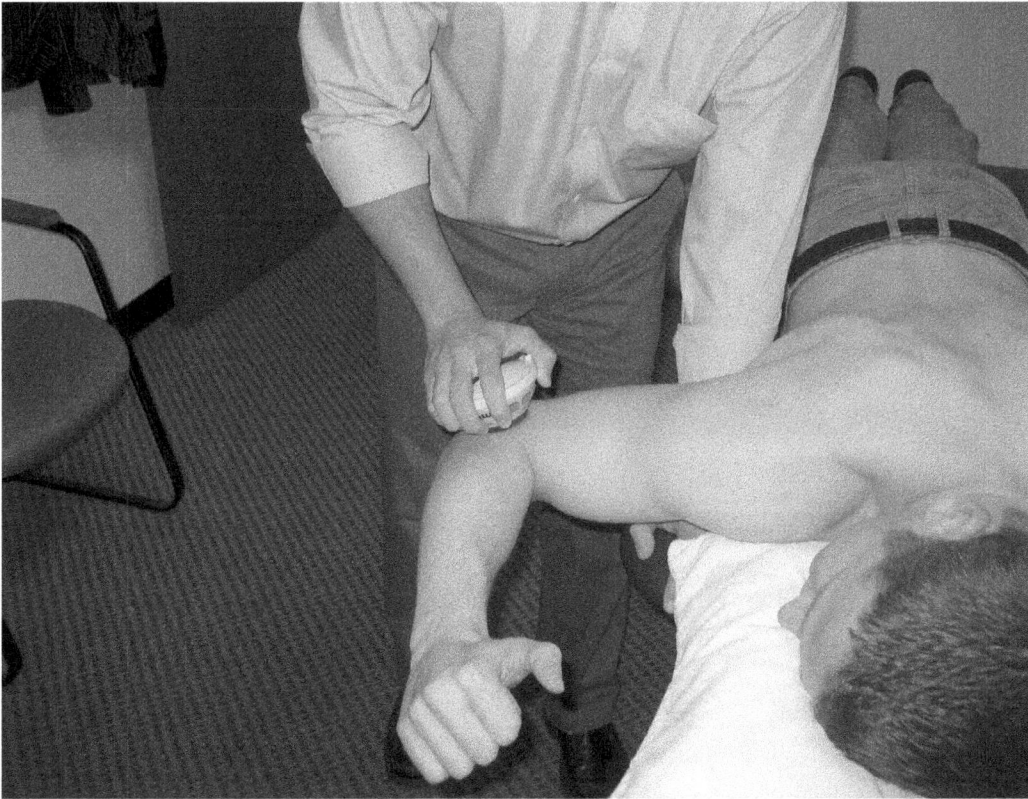

- With the patient in prone, the shoulder is placed in 90° abduction, 90° of lateral rotation and 90° of elbow flexion.
- The patient is instructed to resist the examiner's downward pressure to the lateral elbow directed toward the table and forward. Ekstrom et. al reported that while this movement does not totally isolate the lower traps from the middle and upper traps, it does get the greatest amount of lower trap fibers to fire.

Treatment: If weak, strengthen this muscle with the exercises on pages 49, 51, 59.

Ekstrom RA, Donatelli RA, Soderberg GL. Surface electromyographic analysis of exercises for the trapezius and serratus anterior muscles. *J Orthop Sports Phys Ther.* 33:247-258, 2008.

Mid Trapezius

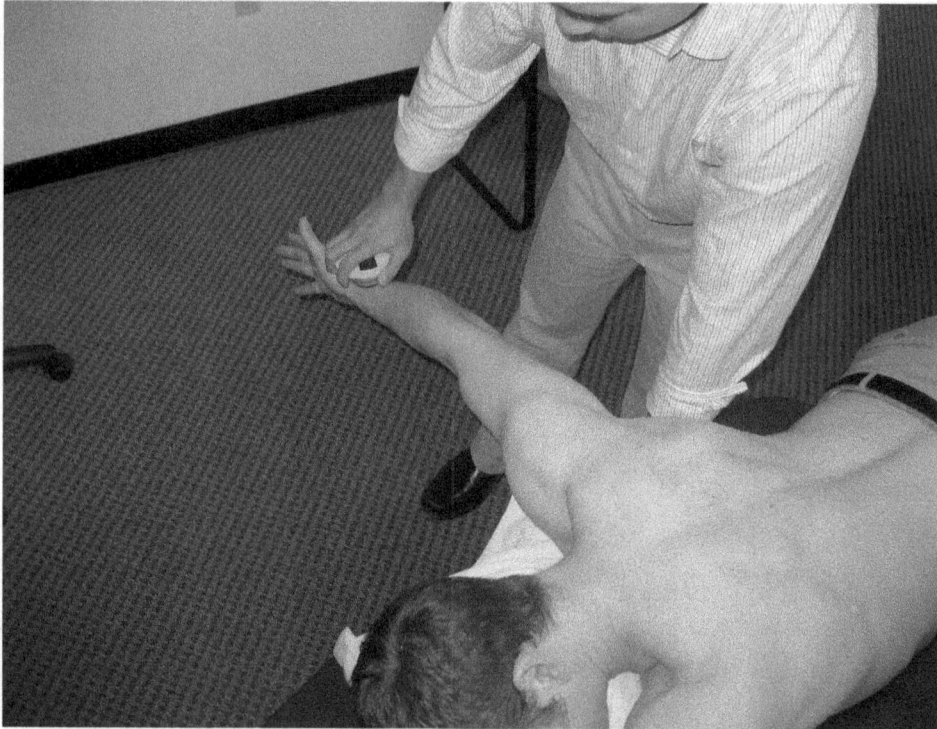

- With the patient in prone, the shoulder is placed in 90° abduction and lateral rotation of the humerus.
- The patient is instructed to resist downward pressure provided by the examiner towards horizontal adduction.
- Mosely et al found maximum EMG activity in the middle trapezius during horizontal abduction with neutral or lateral rotation. Lateral rotation minimizes the contribution from the elbow extensors.

Treatment: If weak, strengthen this muscle with the exercises on pages 47, 49, 50,59,60,66.

Ekstrom RA, Donatelli RA, Soderberg GL. Surface electromyographic analysis of exercises for the trapezius and serratus anterior muscles. *J Orthop Sports Phys Ther.* 33:247-258, 2008. Mosely BJ, et al. EMG analysis of the scapular muscles during a shoulder rehabilitation program. *Am J Sports Med.* 20:128, 1992.

Teres Major

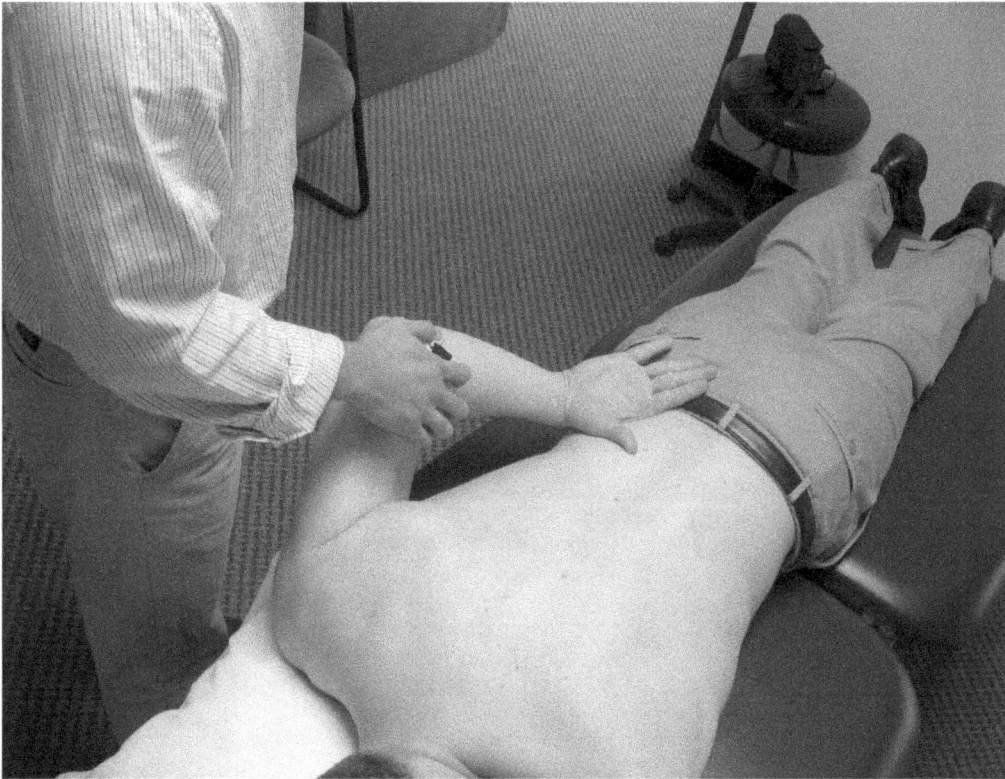

- With the patient in prone, the shoulder is placed in medial rotation with the hand resting on the posterior iliac crest.
- The patient resists as the examiner applies a force above the elbow in the direction of abduction and flexion.

Treatment: If weak, strengthen this muscle with the exercises on page 47.

Kendall FP, McCreary EK, Provance PG. *Muscles: Testing and Function*. Baltimore, MD: Williams and Wilkins; 1993

Latissimus Dorsi

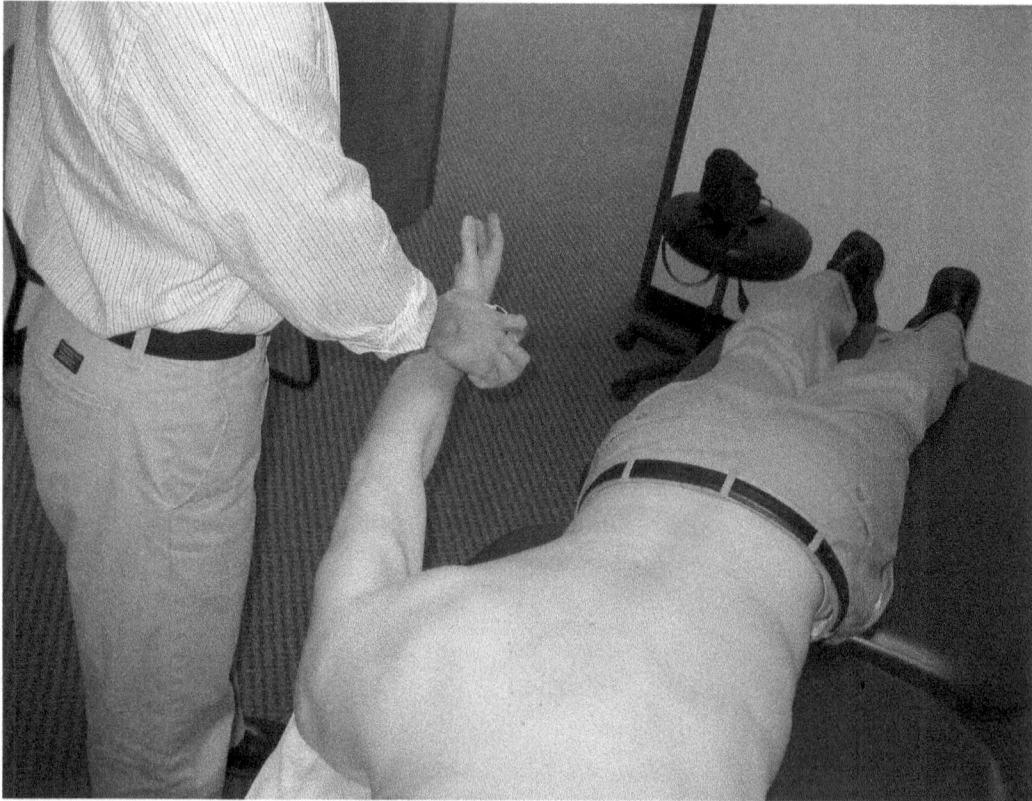

- With the patient in prone, the shoulder is placed in extension, adduction and medial rotation.
- The patient resists as the examiner applies a force against the forearm in the direction of abduction and slight flexion.

Treatment: If weak, strengthen this muscle with the exercises on pages 47, 58.

Kendall FP, McCreary EK, Provance PG. *Muscles: Testing and Function*. Baltimore, MD: Williams and Wilkins; 1993

Rhomboids

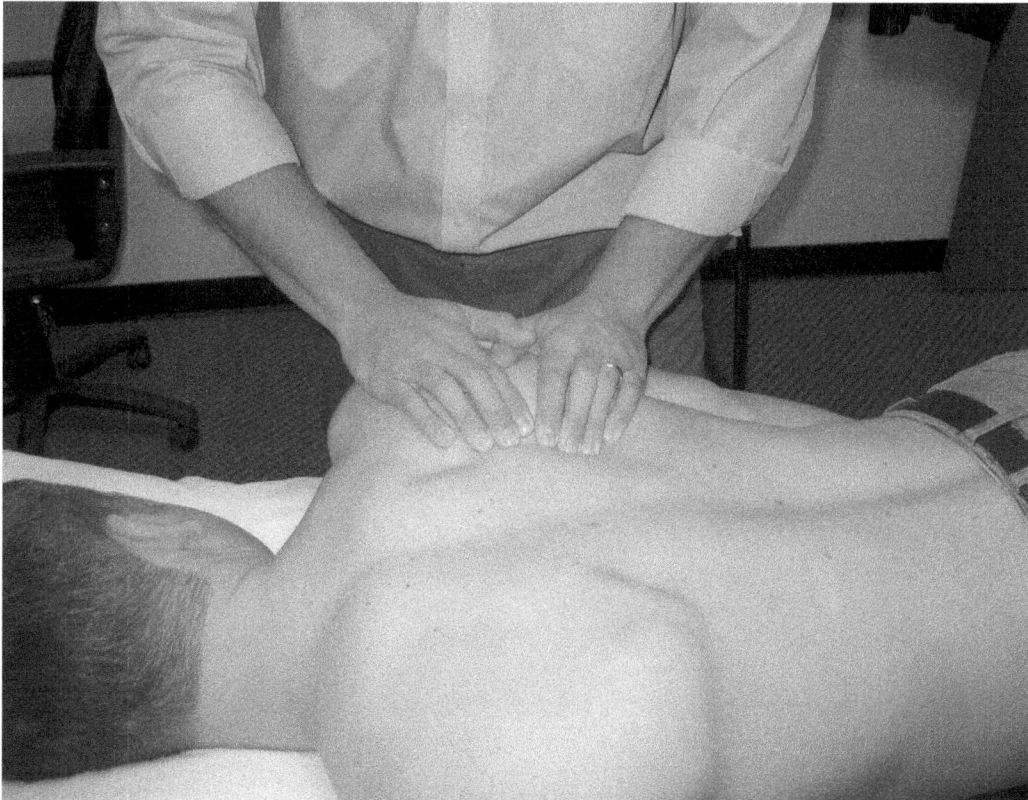

- The patient is placed in prone with arm resting at side.
- The patient resists as the examiner attempts to pull the lateral border of the scapula away from the spine into abduction.

<u>Treatment:</u> If weak, strengthen this muscle with the exercises on pages 47, 49,50,59,60.

Kendall FP, McCreary EK, Provance PG. *Muscles: Testing and Function.* Baltimore, MD: Williams and Wilkins; 1993

Teres Minor

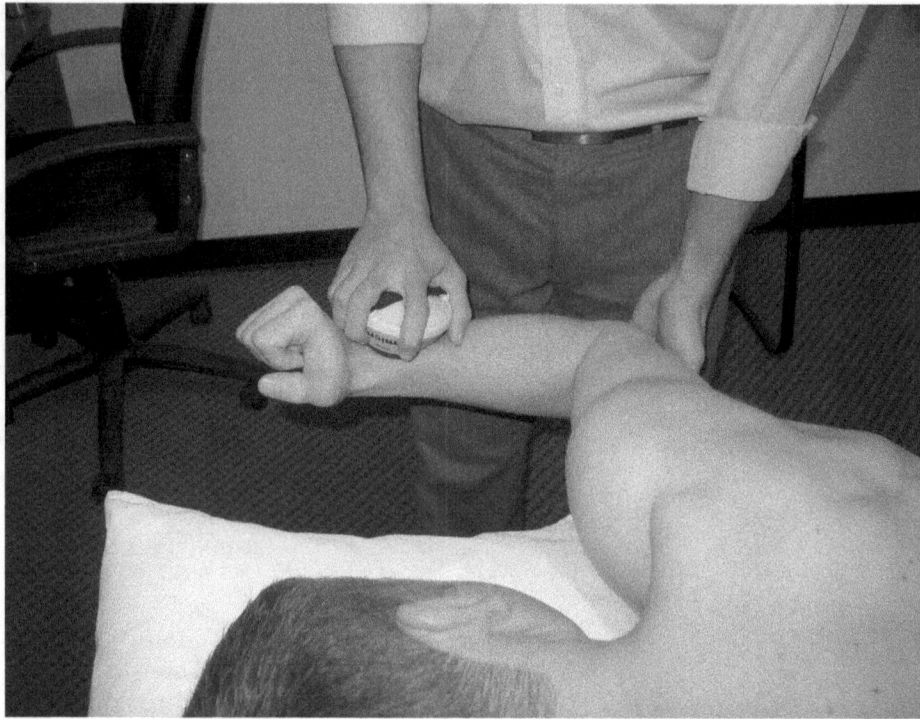

- With the patient prone, the shoulder is placed in 90° abduction, 90° external rotation with elbow bent to 90°.
- The examiner places one hand under the elbow to ensure pure rotation through the humerus. Using the forearm as a lever, pressure is applied in the direction of medial rotation as the patient resists.

Treatment: If weak, strengthen this muscle with the exercises on pages 50,52,53,59,60,61,66.

Kendall FP, McCreary EK, Provance PG. *Muscles: Testing and Function*. Baltimore, MD: Williams and Wilkins; 1993

Special Tests
Impingement Tests
Hawkins Kennedy

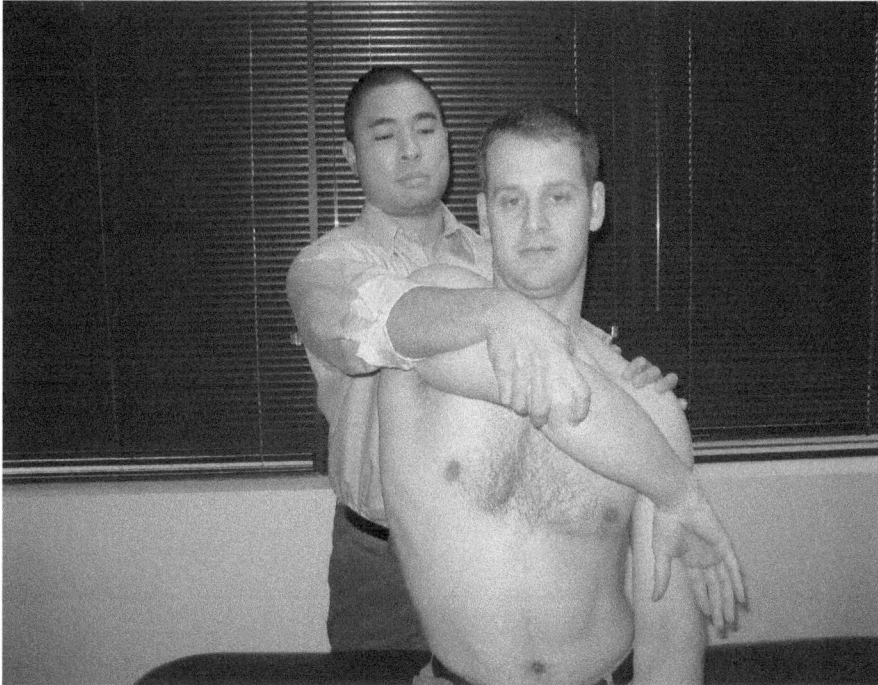

- The examiner forward flexes the arm to 90° and then forcibly medially rotates the shoulder.
- This movement pushes the supraspinatus tendon against the anterior surface of the coracoacromial ligament and coracoid process.
- Pain indicates a positive test for supraspinatus tendinosis or secondary impingement.

Magee DJ. *Orthopedic Physical Assessment*. 4th ed. 2002, Philadelphia: Saunders

Neer's

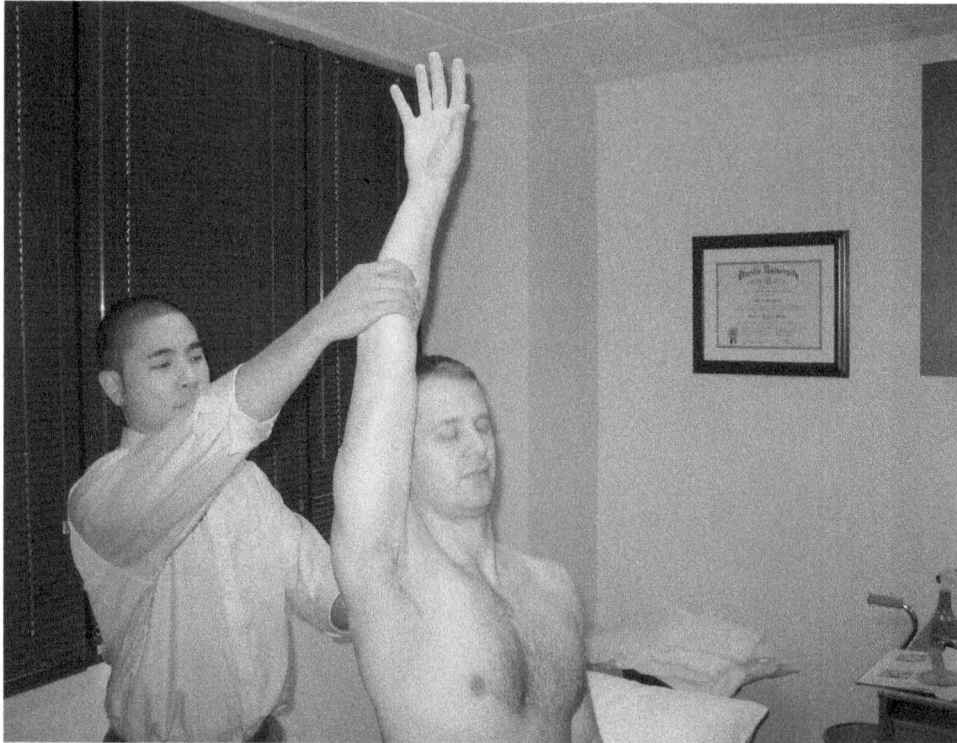

- The patient's arm is passively and forcibly fully elevated in the scapular plane with the arm medially rotated by the examiner.
- A positive Neer impingement sign is present if pain is produced when the arm is forcibly flexed, jamming the greater tuberosity against the anteroinferior border of the acromion.

Magee DJ. *Orthopedic Physical Assessment*. 4th ed. 2002, Philadelphia: Saunders

Yocum

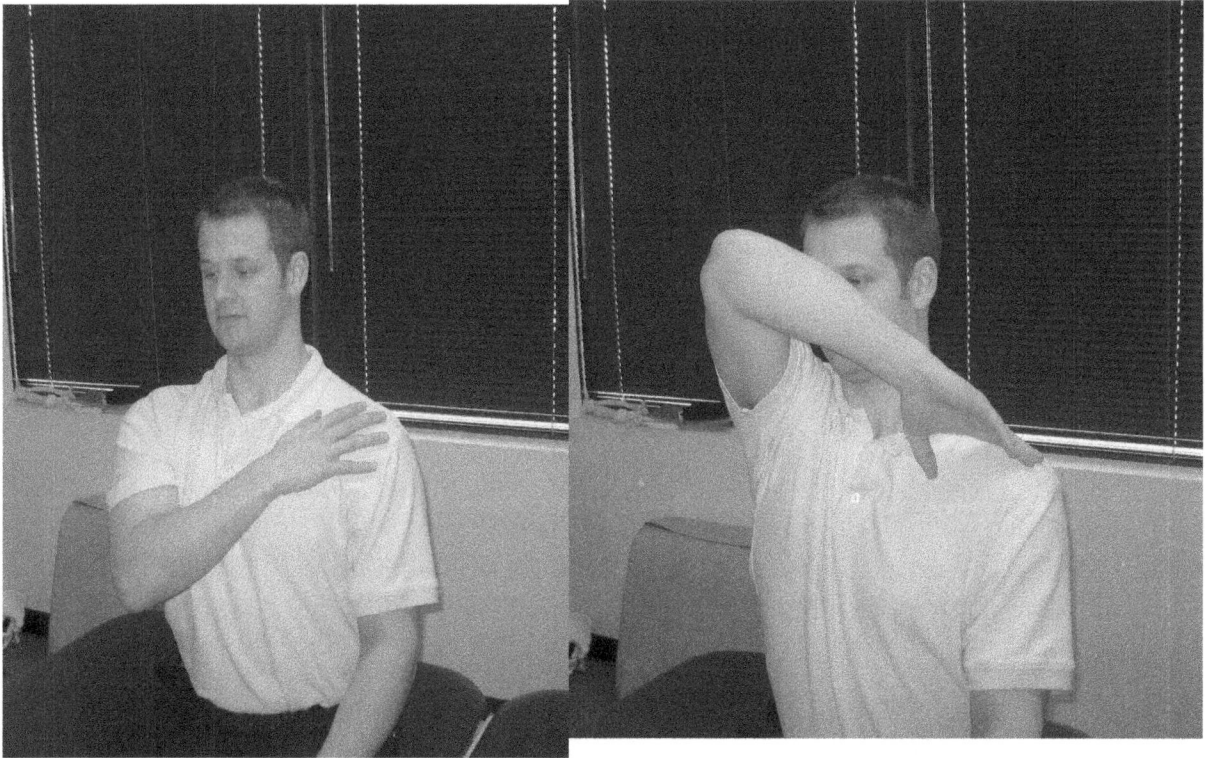

- The patient's hand is placed on the opposite shoulder and the elbow is elevated actively by the patient.
- Pain indicates a positive test for supraspinatus tendinosis or secondary impingement.

Magee DJ. *Orthopedic Physical Assessment*. 4th ed. 2002, Philadelphia: Saunders

Laxity / Instability Tests

Apprehension / Relocation Tests

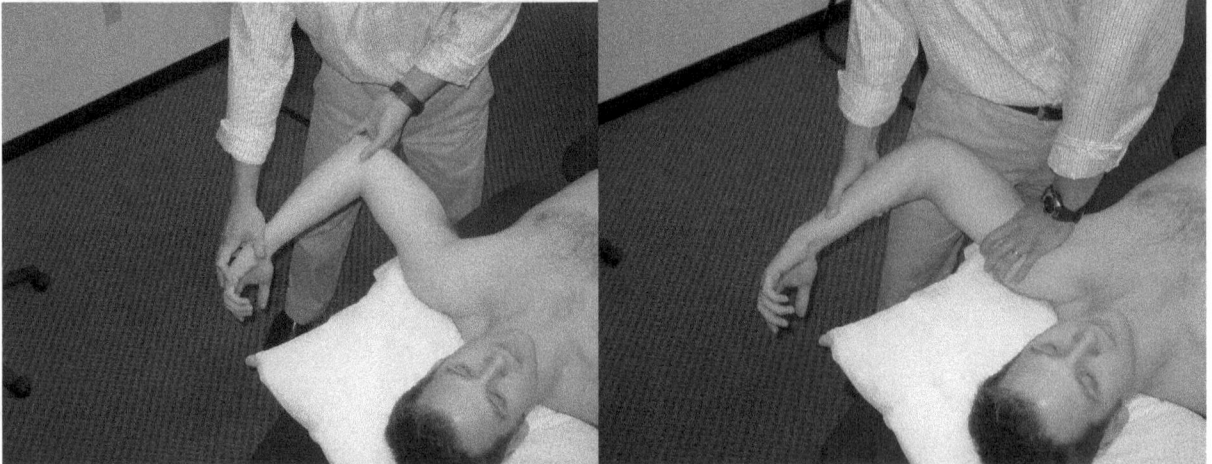

- The examiner abducts the arm to 90° and laterally rotates the patient's shoulder slowly.
- A positive test is indicated by a look or feeling of apprehension or alarm on the patient's face and the patient's resistance to further motion.
- If the Apprehension Test is positive, the examiner then applies a posterior translation stress to the head of the humerus (Relocation Test).
- The test is considered positive if the patient loses the apprehension, pain decreases, and further lateral rotation is possible before the apprehension and/or pain returns.
- These tests are primarily designed to test for traumatic instability problems causing gross or anatomic instability of the shoulder.

Hawkins RJ, Mohtadi NG. Clinical evaluation of shoulder instability. *Clin. J. Sports Med.* 1:59-64, 1991
Magee DJ. *Orthopedic Physical Assessment.* 4th ed. 2002, Philadelphia: Saunders

Sulcus Sign

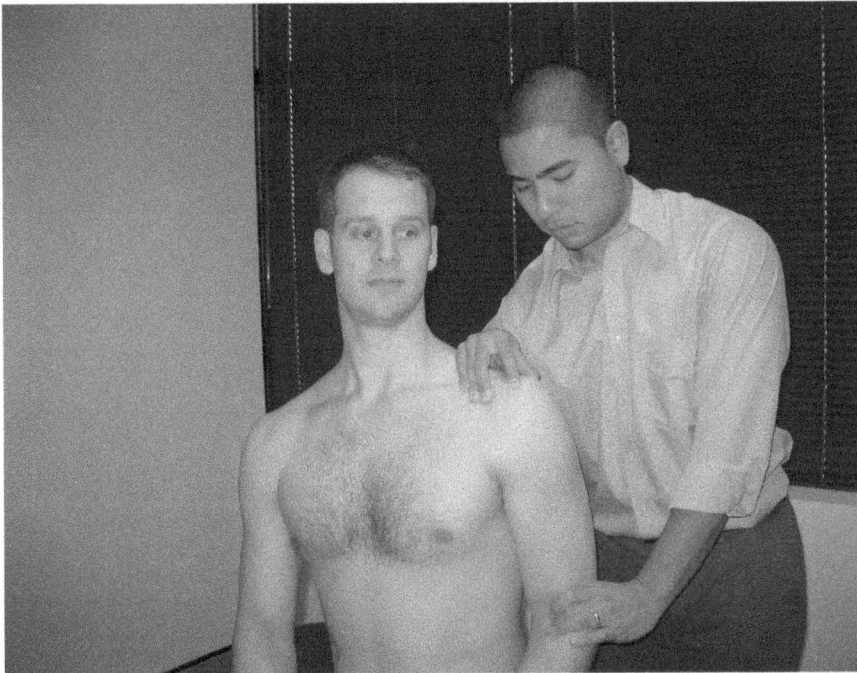

- The patient sits with arm by the side and shoulder muscles relaxed.
- The examiner grasps the patient's forearm below the elbow and pulls the arm distally while palpating the inferior margin of the acromion for inferior translation of the humeral head.
- Presence of a sulcus is considered a positive test and may be indicative of inferior instability or inferior glenohumeral ligament laxity.

Magee DJ. *Orthopedic Physical Assessment*. 4th ed. 2002, Philadelphia: Saunders

Load and Shift

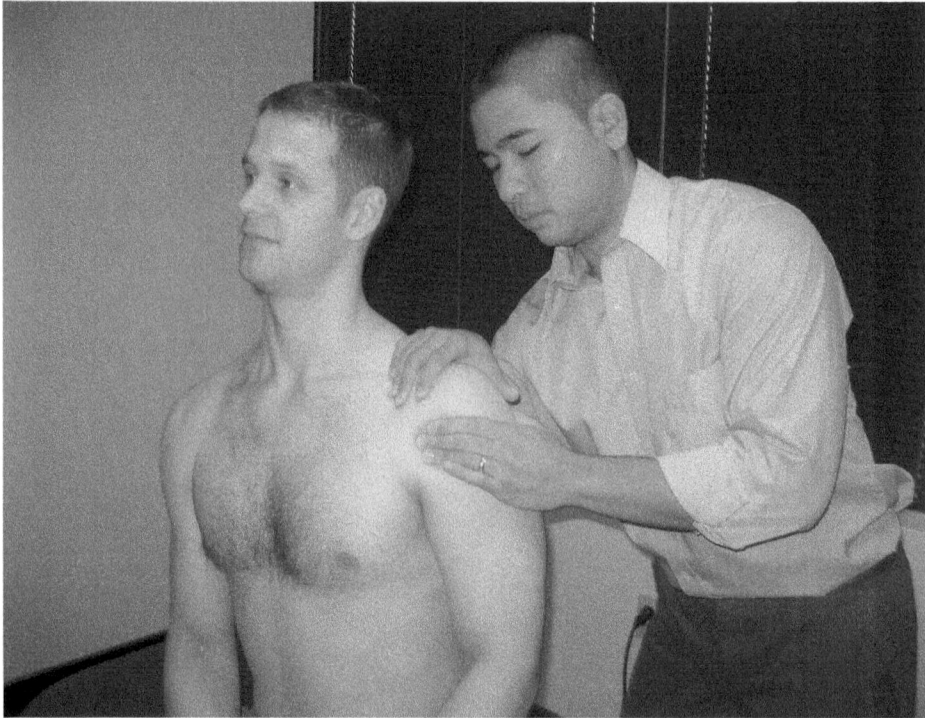

- The patient sits with upright posture with arm at side and shoulder muscles relaxed.
- The examiner stabilizes the shoulder with one hand over the clavicle and scapula.
- With the other hand, the examiner grasps the head of the humerus with the thumb over the posterior humeral head and fingers along the anterior humerus.
- The examiner assesses the initial position of the humeral head relative to the glenoid.
- The humerus is then gently pushed anteriorly or posteriorly to "seat" it into a centered position relative to the glenoid. This is the "load portion" of the test.
- The examiner then pushes the humeral head anteriorly or posteriorly noting the amount of translation and end feel. This is the "shift" portion of the test.

- Translation of 25% or less, of the humeral head diameter anteriorly, is considered normal, although there is variability between patients. Hawkins and Mohtadi advocate a three-grade system for anterior translation.
  - Grade I: the humeral head translates up to 50% riding up to the glenoid rim.
  - Grade II: the humeral head translates more than 50% over the glenoid rim, but spontaneously reduces.
  - Grade III: the humeral head rides over the glenoid rim and does not spontaneously reduce and remains dislocated.

Crank Test

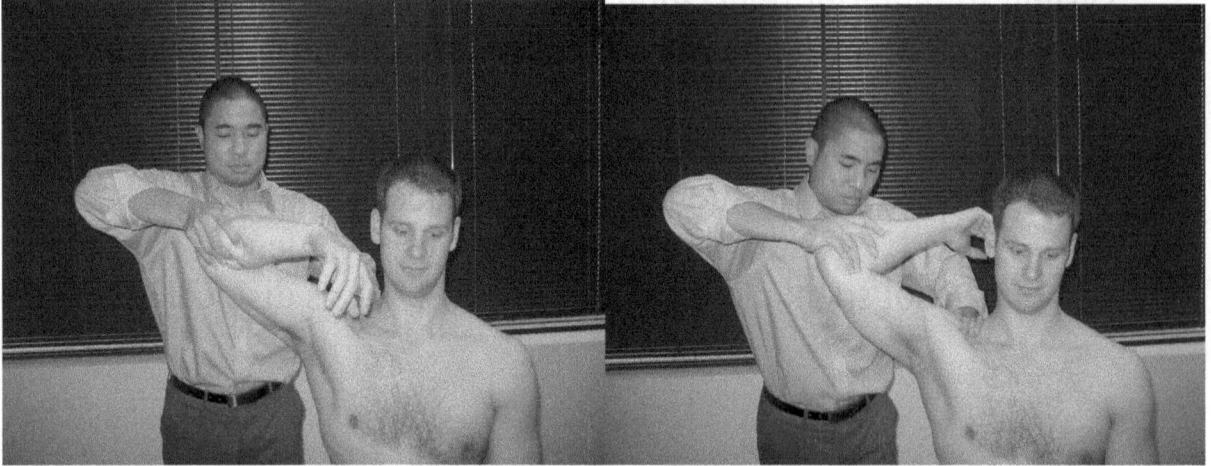

- The patient is in the supine lying or sitting position.
- The examiner elevates the arm to 160° in the scapular plane.
- In this position, an axial load is applied to the humerus with one hand of the examiner while the other hand rotates the humerus medially and laterally.
- A positive test is indicated by pain on rotation. Symptomatic clicking or grinding may also be present during this maneuver.

Magee DJ. *Orthopedic Physical Assessment*. 4th ed. 2002, Philadelphia: Saunders

Wilk KE, et al. Current concepts in the recognition and treatment of superior labral (SLAP) lesions. *Journal of Orthopaedic and Sports Physical Therapy*, 35(5): 273–291, 2005

Active compression Test of O'Brien

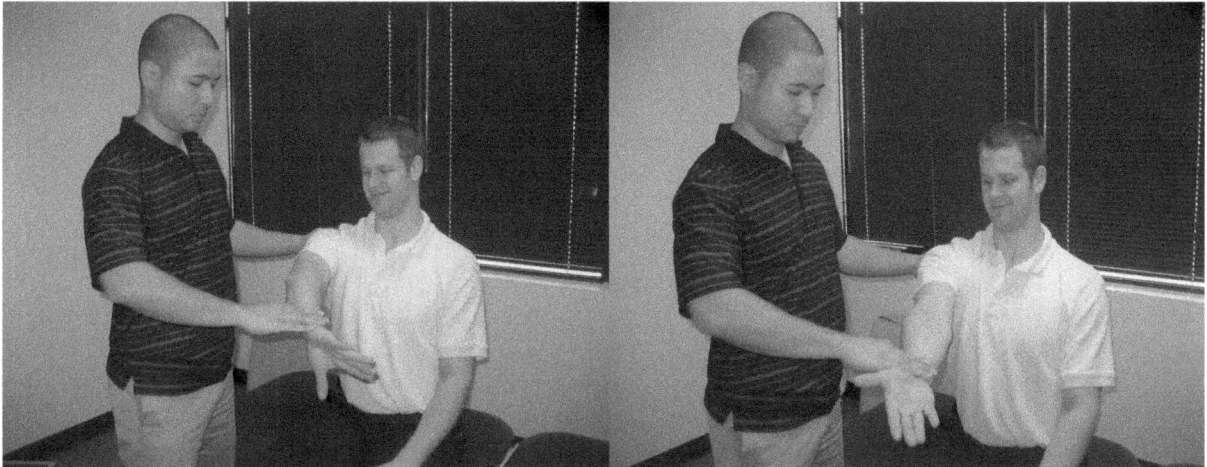

- The patient is placed in the standing position with the arm forward flexed to 90° and the elbow in full extension.
- The arm is then horizontally adducted 10° to 15° and medially rotated so the thumb faces downward.
- The examiner stands beside the patient and applies a downward force to the distal arm.
- With the arm in the same position, the palm is fully supinated and the downward force is repeated.
- The test is considered positive for labral abnormality if pain and/or clicking are produced "inside" the shoulder with the first maneuver and reduced or eliminated with the second maneuver.
- Pain localized to the acromioclavicular joint or on top of the shoulder is diagnostic of acromioclavicular joint abnormality.

O'Brien SJ, Pagnani MJ, Fealy S, et al: The active compression test: A new and effective test for diagnosing labral tears and acromioclavicular joint abnormality. *Am J Sports Med* 26:610-613, 1998

Magee DJ. *Orthopedic Physical Assessment*. 4th ed. 2002, Philadelphia: Saunders

New Pain Provocation Test

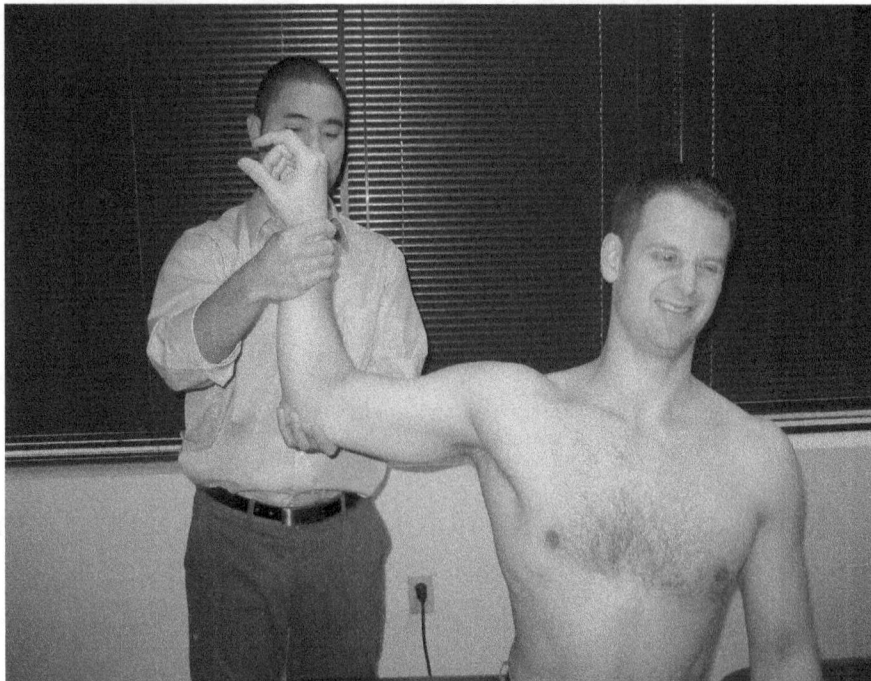

- The patient is seated and the arm is abducted to between 90° and 100° and the arm is laterally rotated by the examiner by holding the wrist.
- The forearm is taken into maximum supination, and then maximum pronation. If pain is provoked only in the pronated position, the test is considered positive for a SLAP tear.
- In this position, forearm pronation produces additional stretch to the biceps tendon.

Magee DJ. *Orthopedic Physical Assessment*. 4th ed. 2002, Philadelphia: Saunders
Mimori K, Menta T, Nakagawa T, Shinomiya K. A new pain provocation test for superior labral tears of the shoulder. *Am J Sports Med*, 27(2):137-142, 1999

Bicep Load Test II

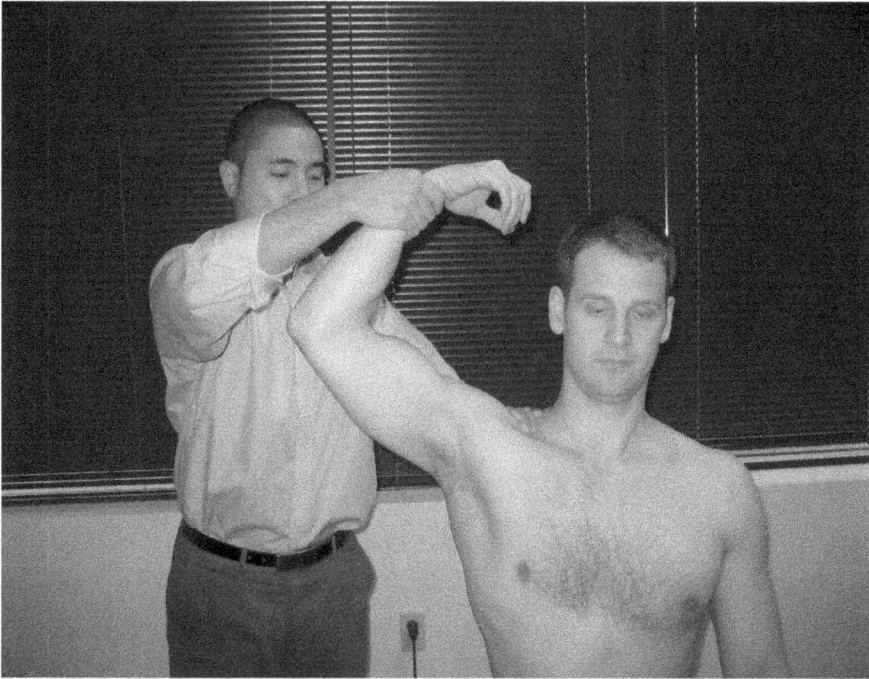

- The arm to be examined is elevated to 120° (can also elevate to 90 deg) and laterally rotated to its maximal point with the elbow in 90° flexion and the forearm in the supinated position.
- The patient is asked to flex the elbow while resisting the examiner's resistance at the wrist.
- The test is considered positive if the patient complains of increased pain during the resisted elbow flexion.
- The test is negative if pain is not elicited by the resisted elbow flexion or if the preexisting pain during the elevation and external rotation of the arm is unchanged or diminished by the resisted elbow flexion.

Kim SH, Ha KI, Ahn JH, et al: Biceps load test II: A clinical test for SLAP lesions of the shoulder. *Arthroscopy* 17: 160-164, 2001
Magee DJ. *Orthopedic Physical Assessment*. 4th ed. 2002, Philadelphia: Saunders

Speeds Test

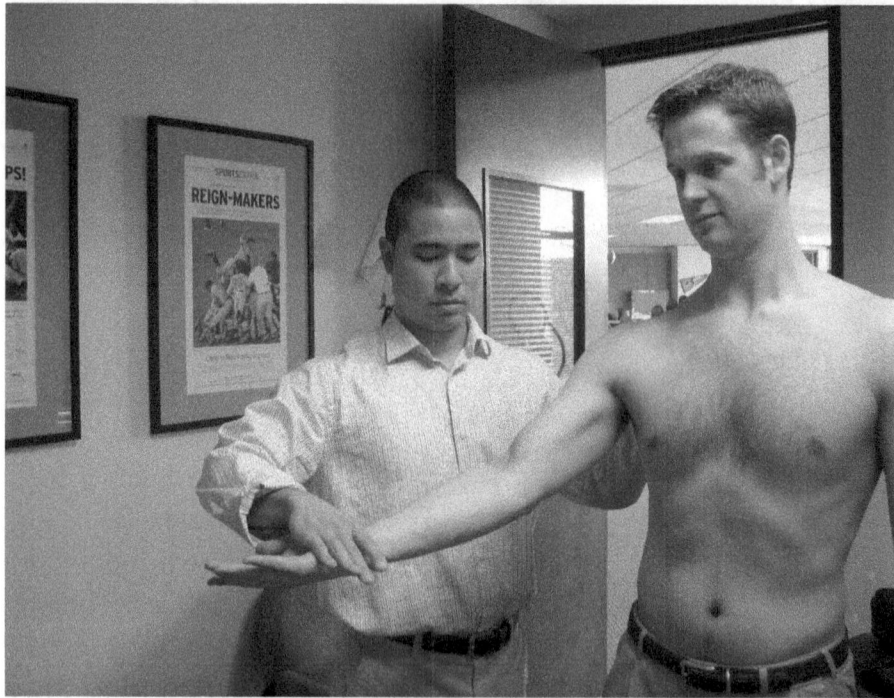

- The patient resists downward force with shoulder flexed to 90° and elbow fully extended.
- A positive test elicits increased tenderness in the biciptal groove and is indicative of a SLAP lesion or bicipital tendinosis.

Magee DJ. *Orthopedic Physical Assessment*. 4th ed. 2002, Philadelphia: Saunders

Wilk KE, et al. Current concepts in the recognition and treatment of superior labral (SLAP) lesions. *Journal of Orthopaedic and Sports Physical Therapy*, 35(5): 273–291, 2005

Dynamic Speeds Tests

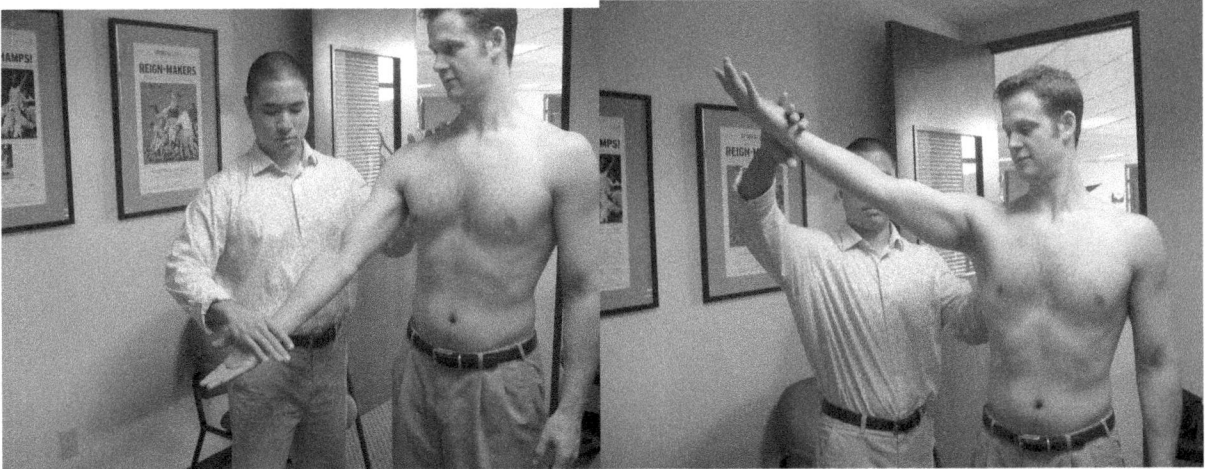

- The examiner provides resistance against both shoulder elevation and elbow flexion simultaneously as the patient elevates the arm overhead.
- Deep pain within the shoulder is with shoulder elevation is positive for labral pathology

Magee DJ. *Orthopedic Physical Assessment*. 4th ed. 2002, Philadelphia: Saunders

Wilk KE, et al. Current concepts in the recognition and treatment of superior labral (SLAP) lesions. *Journal of Orthopaedic and Sports Physical Therapy*, 35(5): 273–291, 2005

Rotator Cuff Pathology Tests

Bear Hug

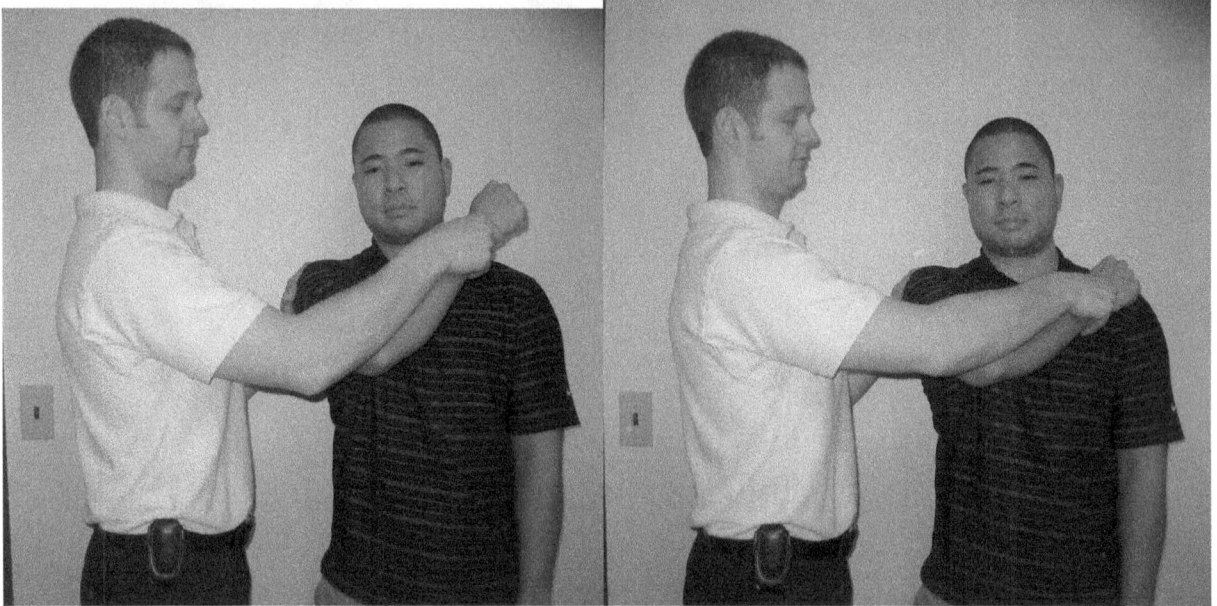

- The patient's fist is placed on their opposite shoulder
- The therapist tries to lift the patient's wrist off their opposite shoulder while the patient resists.
- Inability to hold the position due to weakness or pain may indicate a lesion of the subscapularis muscle or tendon.

Johannes RH, et al. the Bear Hug Test: A New and Sensitive Test for Diagnosing a Subscapularis Tear. *Arthroscopy: The Journal of Arthroscopic and Related Surgery*, 22(10):1076-1084, 2006

Internal Rotation Lag Sign

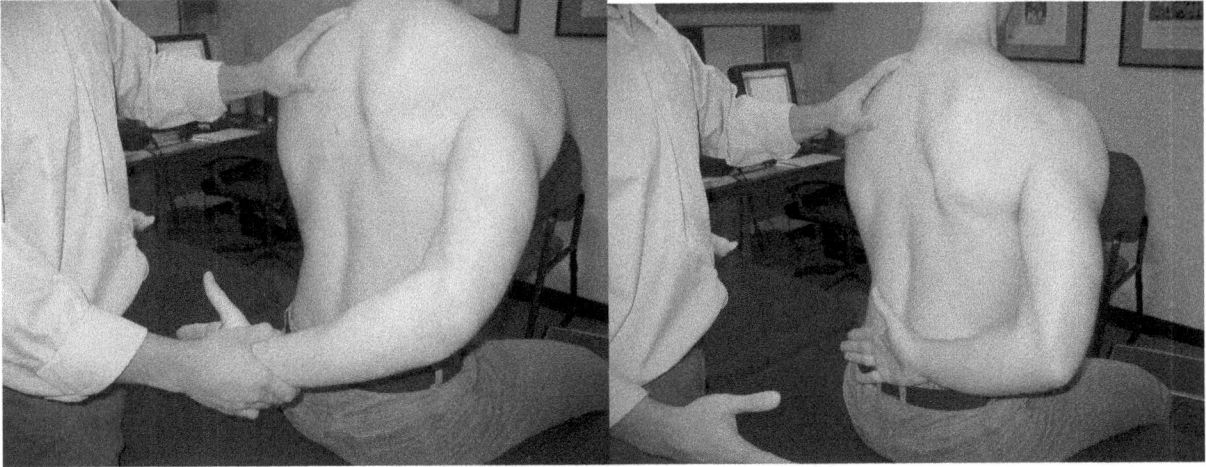

- The patient's hand is passively medially rotated and brought behind the back as far as possible.
- The elbow is flexed at 90°, and the shoulder is held at 20° elevation and 20° extension.
- The patient is then asked to hold the position as the examiner releases the wrist while maintaining support at the elbow.
- The sign is considered positive when a lag occurs and the patient is unable to maintain maximum internal rotation and the hand moves toward the back.
- Inability to hold the position due to weakness or pain may indicate a lesion of the subscapularis muscle or tendon.

Magee DJ. *Orthopedic Physical Assessment*. 4th ed. 2002, Philadelphia: Saunders
Tennent TD, Beach WR, Meyers J. Clinical Sports Medicine Update. A Review of the Special Tests Associated with Shoulder Examination: Part I: The Rotator Cuff Tests
Am. J. Sports Med. 31: 154 – 160, 2003

ERLS (Lag sign for tear of supraspinatus / infraspinatus)

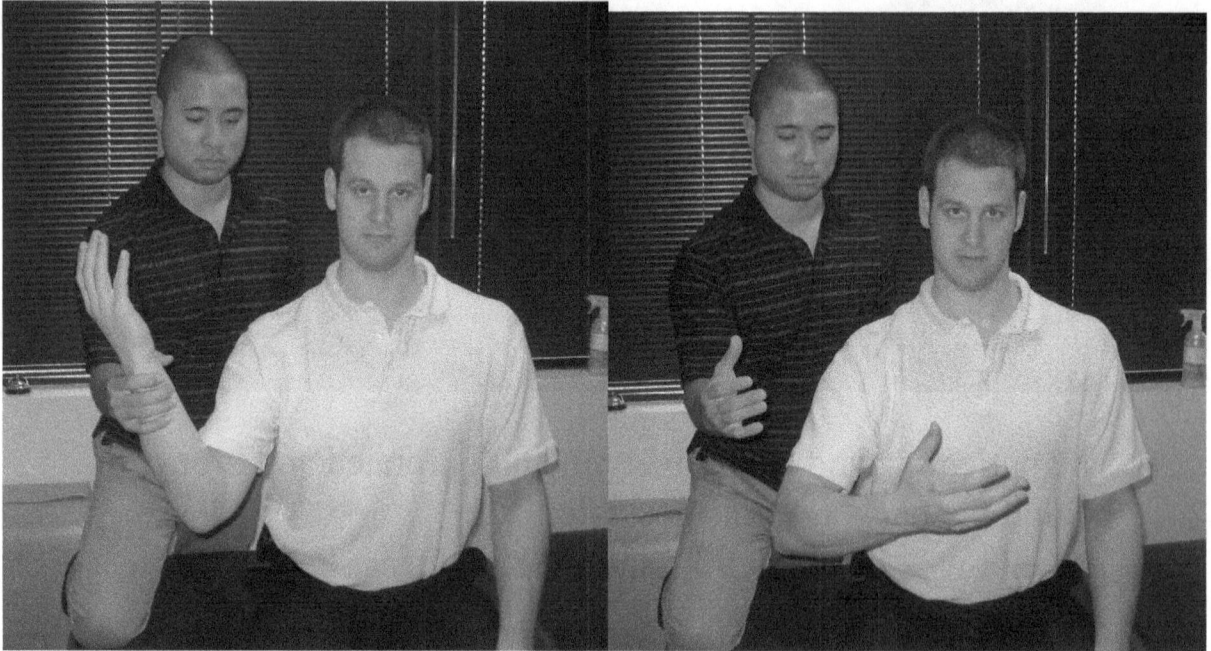

- The patient's elbow is passively flexed to 90° and the shoulder is held at 20° elevation in the scapular plane.
- The examiner then takes the patient's arm into maximum lateral rotation and asks the patient to hold the position as he releases the wrist while maintaining support at the elbow.
- If the supraspinatus and infraspinatus tendons are torn the arm will medially rotate and spring back anteriorly indicating a positive test.

Magee DJ. *Orthopedic Physical Assessment*. 4th ed. 2002, Philadelphia: Saunders
Tennent TD, Beach WR, Meyers J. Clinical Sports Medicine Update. A Review of the Special Tests Associated with Shoulder Examination: Part I: The Rotator Cuff Tests
Am. J. Sports Med. 31: 154 – 160, 2003

External Rotation Lag Sign (for tear of infraspinatus)

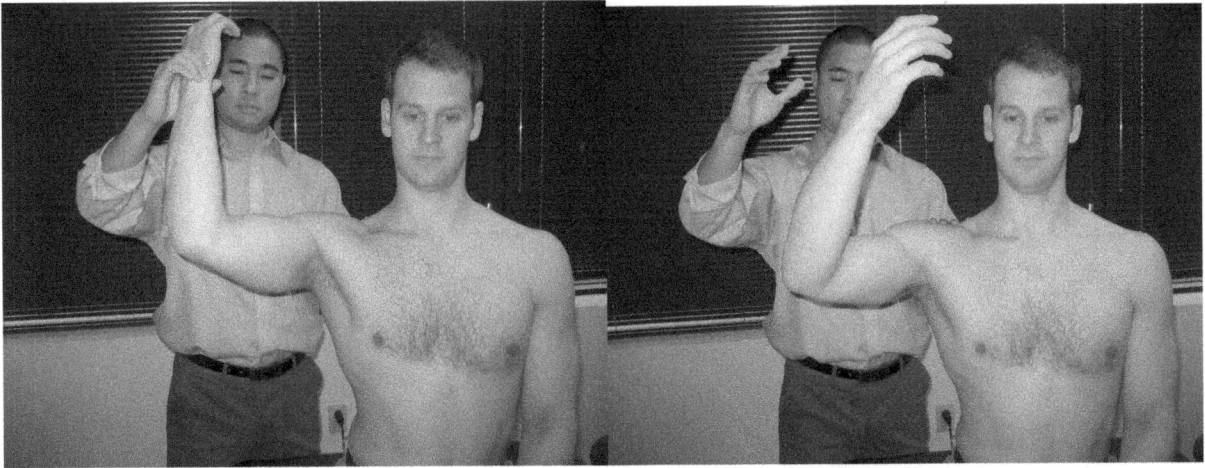

- The examiner holds the affected arm at 90° of elevation in the scapular plane at maximal external rotation with the elbow flexed at 90°.
- The patient is asked to actively maintain this position as the examiner releases the wrist while supporting the elbow.
- If the patient's hand springs forward and "drops" back to neutral rotation the test is considered positive for a lesion of the infraspinatus.

Magee DJ. *Orthopedic Physical Assessment*. 4th ed. 2002, Philadelphia: Saunders
Tennent TD, Beach WR, Meyers J. Clinical Sports Medicine Update. A Review of the Special Tests Associated with Shoulder Examination: Part I: The Rotator Cuff Tests
Am. J. Sports Med. 31: 154 – 160, 2003

Acromioclavicular Shear Test

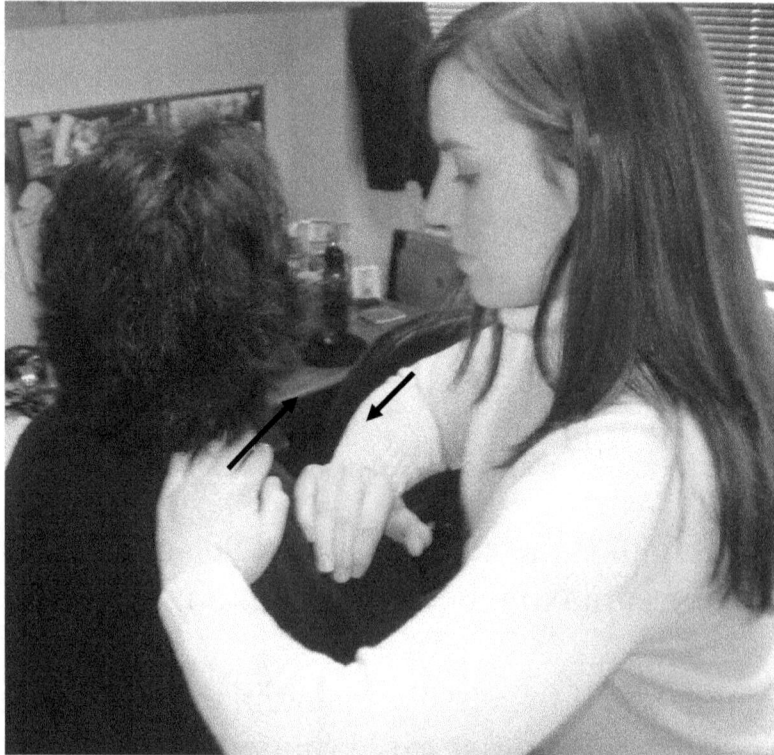

- With the patient in a sitting position, the examiner places one hand over the spine of the scapula and the other on the clavicle.
- The examiner squeezes the hands together.
- A positive test is indicated by pain or abnormal movement at the AC joint.

Magee DJ. *Orthopedic Physical Assessment*. 4th ed. 2002, Philadelphia: Saunders

Mobilizations
Restriction in External Rotation at 0 deg Abduction
Subscapularis Tilt

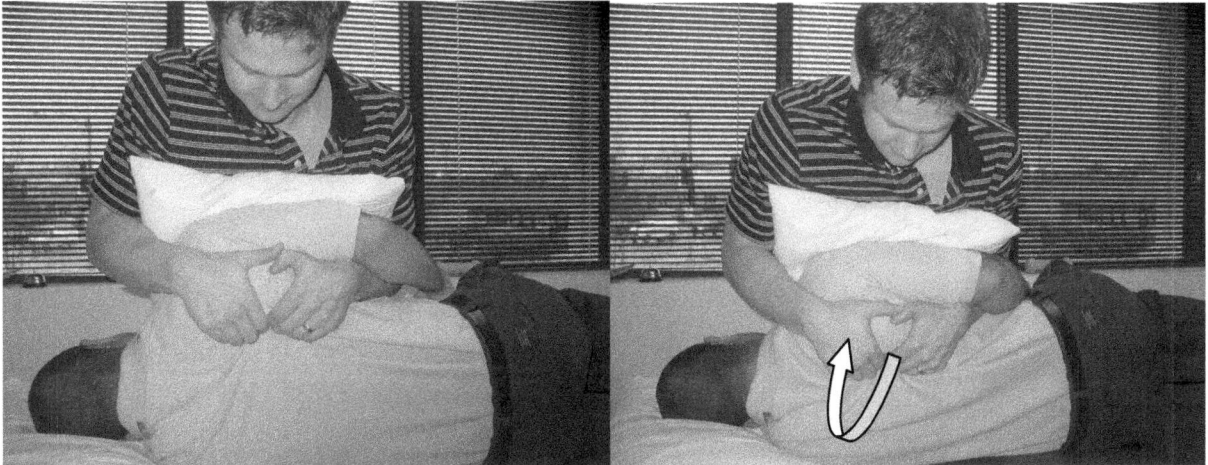

Anterior Approach

- **Patient Position:** Side lying close to the edge of the table, with the involved extremity side up.
- **Therapist Position:**
  - Facing the patient with the caudal hand underneath the inferior angle of the scapula and the cephalad hand grasping the vertebral border of the scapula.
  - The therapist's sternum is the third contact point assisting the scapular tilt. Both hands tilt the scapula away from the thoracic wall.

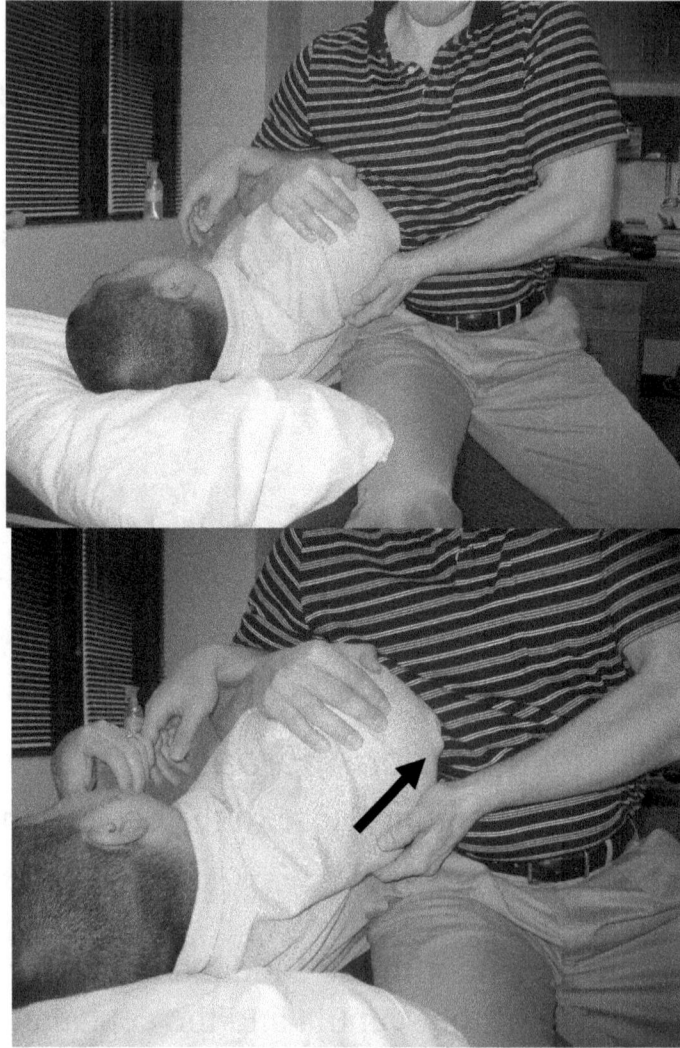

Posterior Approach

- **Patient Position:** Side lying as previous, but closer to the posterior edge of the table.
- **Therapist Position:**
  - Posterior to patient with inner hand thread under the involved extremity and supporting the anterior glenohumeral joint.
  - Outer mobilizing hand grasps the vertebral border and tilts the scapula away from the thoracic wall.

Turkel SJ, Panio MW, Marshall JL, Girgis FG: Stabilizing mechanisms preventing anterior dislocation of the glenohumeral joint. J Bone Joint Surg 63 A: 1208-1217, 1981.
Donatelli RA, *Physical Therapy of the Shoulder*. 4th Ed. 2004, Missouri: Elsevier.

Coracohumeral Ligament Mobilization
(used if the subscapularis tilt does not work)

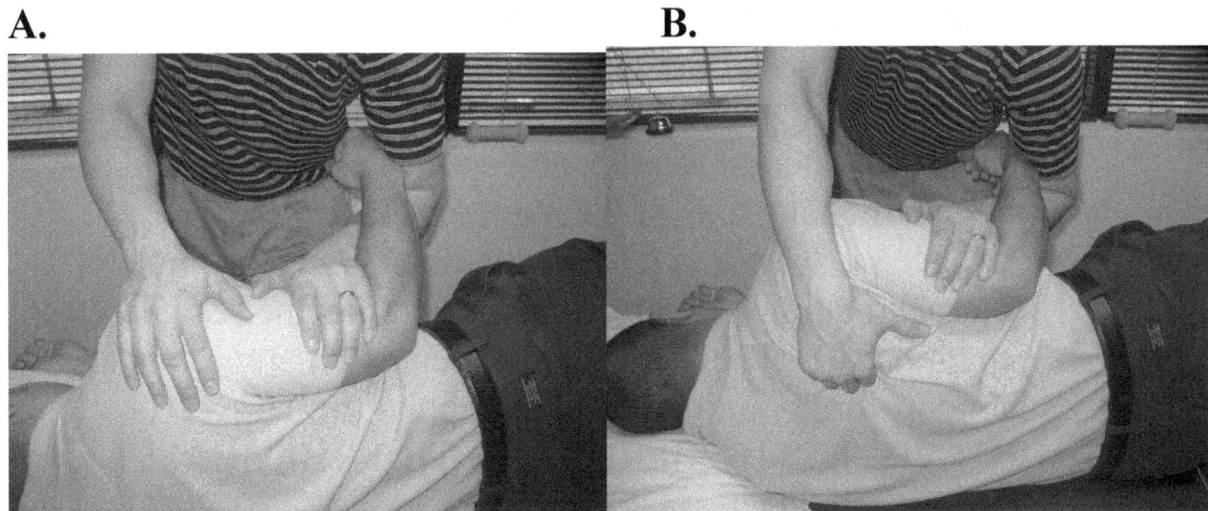

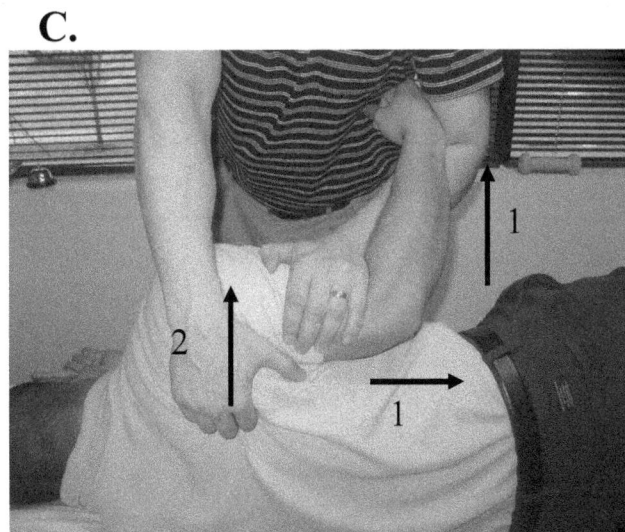

A.

B.

C.

- **Patient Position:** Side lying close to the edge of the table, with the involved extremity side up.
- **Therapist Position:**
  - **A.** Facing the patient with the caudal hand grasping the patient's arm above the elbow while the patient's anterior forearm rests on the therapist's posterior forearm.
  - **B.** The therapist's cephalad hand grasps the vertebral border of the scapula and tilts away from the thoracic wall. If the

therapist is unable to get under the scapula, bring the patient's arm into internal rotation.

- o **C.** Once the therapist's cephalad hand is under the patient's vertebral border of the scapula, the therapist's caudal hand simultaneously takes the patient's arm into the desired amount of external rotation and applies an inferior glide through the long axis of the humerus (1).
- o **C.** Once the barrier is felt; the therapist holds the humeral external rotation and inferior glide and tilts the scapula x 10 repetitions (2). The therapist can then externally rotate the humerus further and repeat the scapular tilt. DO NOT ROTATE THE HUMERUS AND TILT THE SCAPULA AT THE SAME TIME.

Bowen MK, Warren RF: Ligamentous control of shoulder stability based on selective cutting and static translation experiments. Clin Sports Med 10:757-782

Supine Inferior Glide in External Rotation

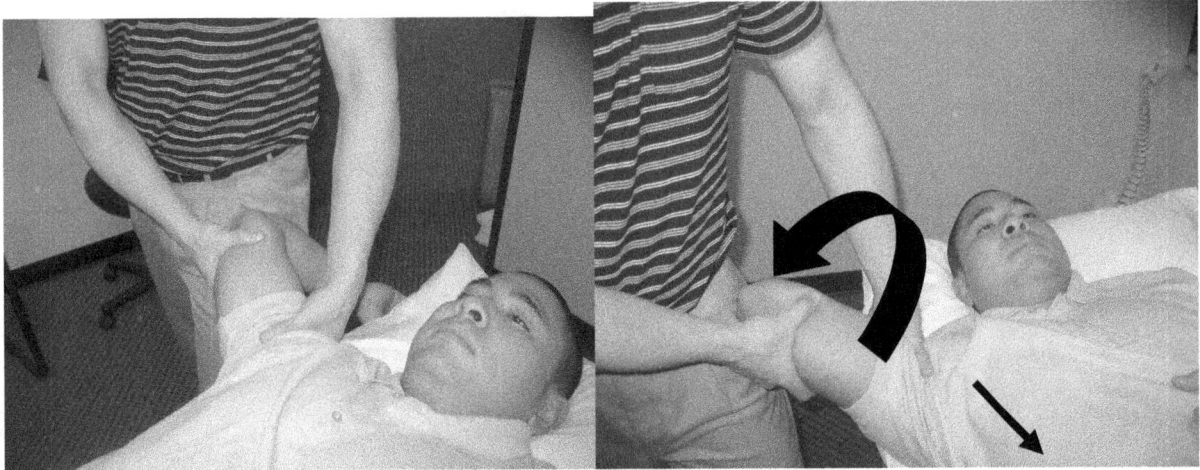

- **Patient Position:** Supine with involved extremity close to the edge of the table.
- **Therapist Position:**
  - Facing the lateral aspect of the patient's upper arm.
  - The patient's arm is taken into 90 deg. of abduction in the scapular plane and externally rotated to the desired range.
  - The therapist's cephalad hand web space is placed on the superior glenohumeral joint inferior to the acromion.
  - The assisting had supports the weight of the arm by holding the distal upper arm while maintaining rotation.
  - The mobilizing hand glides the head of the humerus inferiorly, attempting to stress the inferior fibers of the posterior capsule that have moved inferiorly with external rotation of the humerus.

Donatelli RA, *Physical Therapy of the Shoulder.* 4th ed. 2004, Missouri: Elsevier.
Bowen MK, Warren RF: Ligamentous control of shoulder stability based on selective cutting and static translation experiments. Clin Sports Med 10:757-782

Posterior Capsule Mobilization

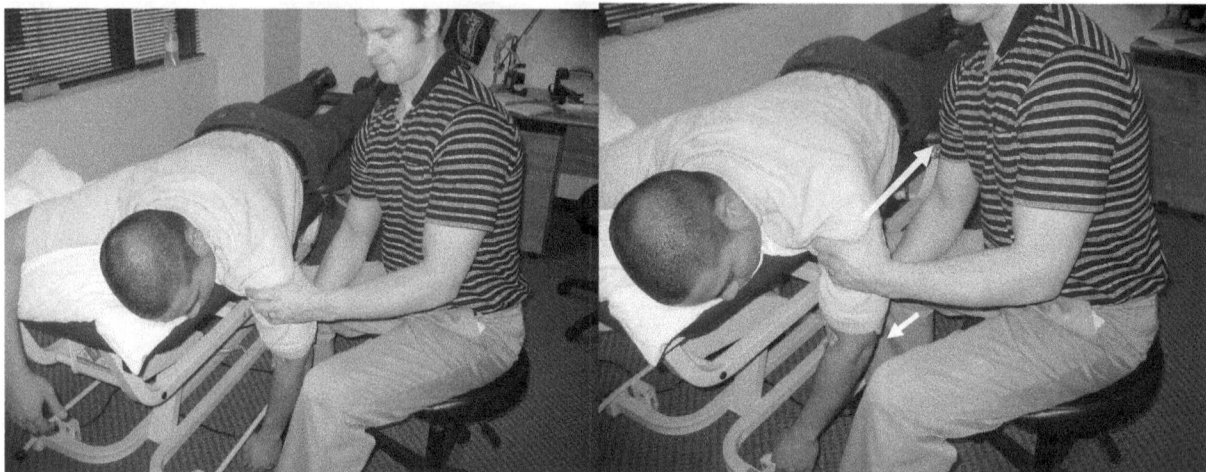

- **Patient Position**: Prone with the involved extremity hanging off the edge of the table.
- **Therapist Position:**
  - Facing the patient in a sitting position, the therapist grasps the humeral head with the cephalad hand and supports the elbow with their caudal hand. Make sure that the therapist's body is lined up to the line of pull for the mobilization.
  - A quick anteroposterior movement is used to oscillate the head of the humerus into the barrier while at the same time the caudal hand moves the elbow anteriorly.

Bowen MK, Warren RF: Ligamentous control of shoulder stability based on selective cutting and static translation experiments. Clin Sports Med 10:757-782

Prone Inferior Glide in External Rotation

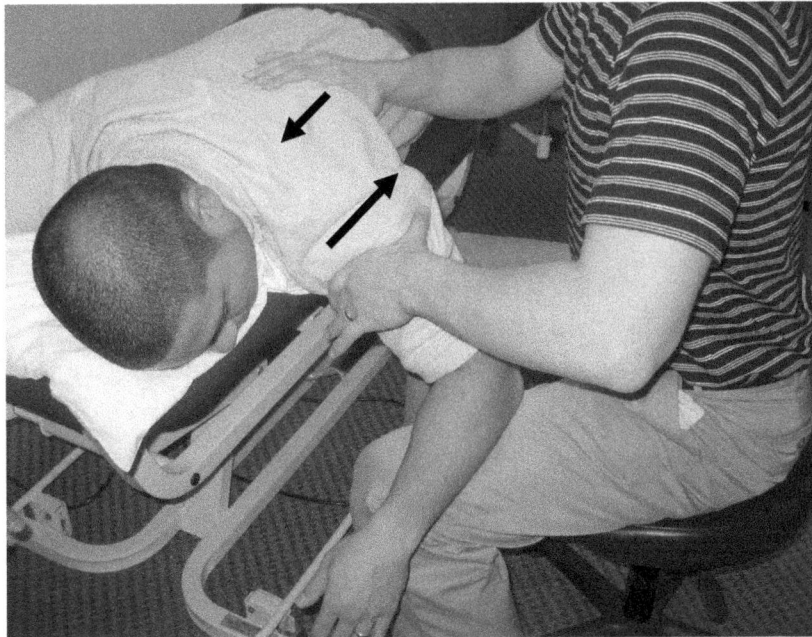

- **Patient Position:** Prone with involved extremity hanging off the edge of the table.
- **Therapist Position:**
  - Seated facing the involved extremity.
  - The patient's medial elbow rests on the therapist's cephalad knee in external rotation and 90 deg. of abduction in the plane of the scapula.
  - The therapists cephalad hand stabilizes the scapula along the lateral border with the thumb blocking the inferior glenoid.
  - The therapist's cephalad hand web space is placed on the superior glenohumeral joint inferior to the acromion.
  - The cephalad hand glides the head of the humerus inferiorly while the caudal hand glides the scapula superiorly.
  - This will stress the inferior band of the posterior capsule that has moved inferiorly with external rotation of the humerus

Bowen MK, Warren RF: Ligamentous control of shoulder stability based on selective cutting and static translation experiments. Clin Sports Med 10:757-782

Prone Internal Rotation Hang

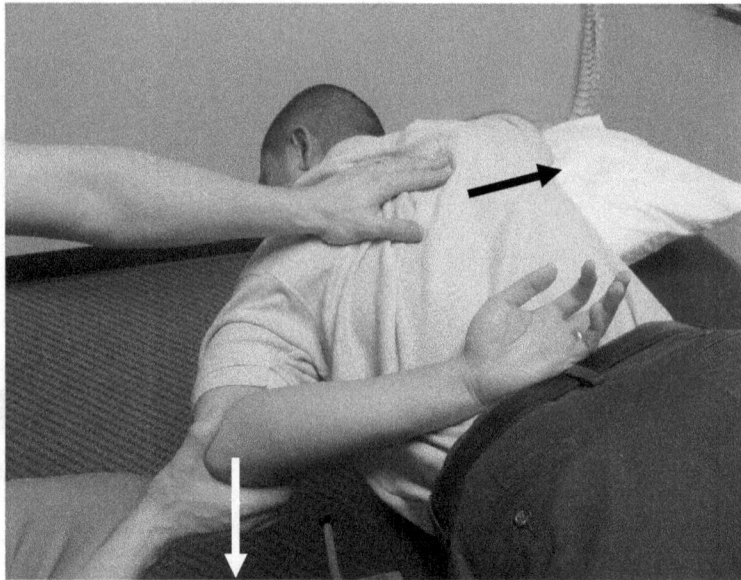

- **Patient Position:** Prone with involved extremity lying next to the patient.
- **Therapist Position:**
  - Seated facing the patient.
  - The patient's hand is placed on their lumbar spine (if patient is unable to internally rotate enough place their hand on the table with the dorsum of the hand on the table and the elbow bent).
  - The therapists cephalad hand stabilizes the scapula along the spinal border.
  - The therapist's caudal hand places a gentle downward force on the patient's medial elbow.
  - Hold for 2-3 minutes, reset and repeat 2-3 times.

Izumi T, Aoki M, et al: Stretching postions for the posterior capsule of the glenohumeral joint. Amer J Sports Med 36: 2014-2022.

Middle Glenohumeral Mobilization

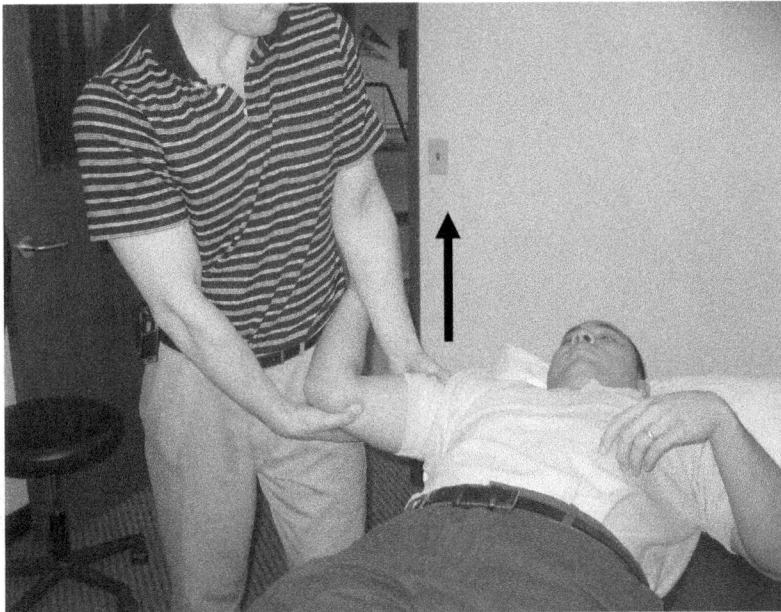

- **Patient Position:** Supine with involved extremity close to the edge of the table.
- **Therapist Position:**
  - Facing the lateral aspect of the patient's upper arm.
  - The patient's arm is taken into 45 deg. of abduction in the scapular plane and externally rotated to the desired range.
  - The therapist's cephalad hand web space is placed on the posterior glenohumeral joint.
  - The assisting had supports the weight of the arm by holding the distal upper arm while maintaining rotation.
  - The mobilizing hand glides the head of the humerus anteriorly, attempting to stress the middle glenohumeral ligament.

Turkel SJ, Panio MW, Marshall JL, Girgis FG: Stabilizing mechanisms preventing anterior dislocation of the glenohumeral joint. J Bone Joint Surg 63 A: 1208-1217, 1981.
Donatelli RA, *Physical Therapy of the Shoulder.* 4th ed. 2004, Missouri: Elsevier.

Fulcrum Technique
(To mobilize the posterior capsule)

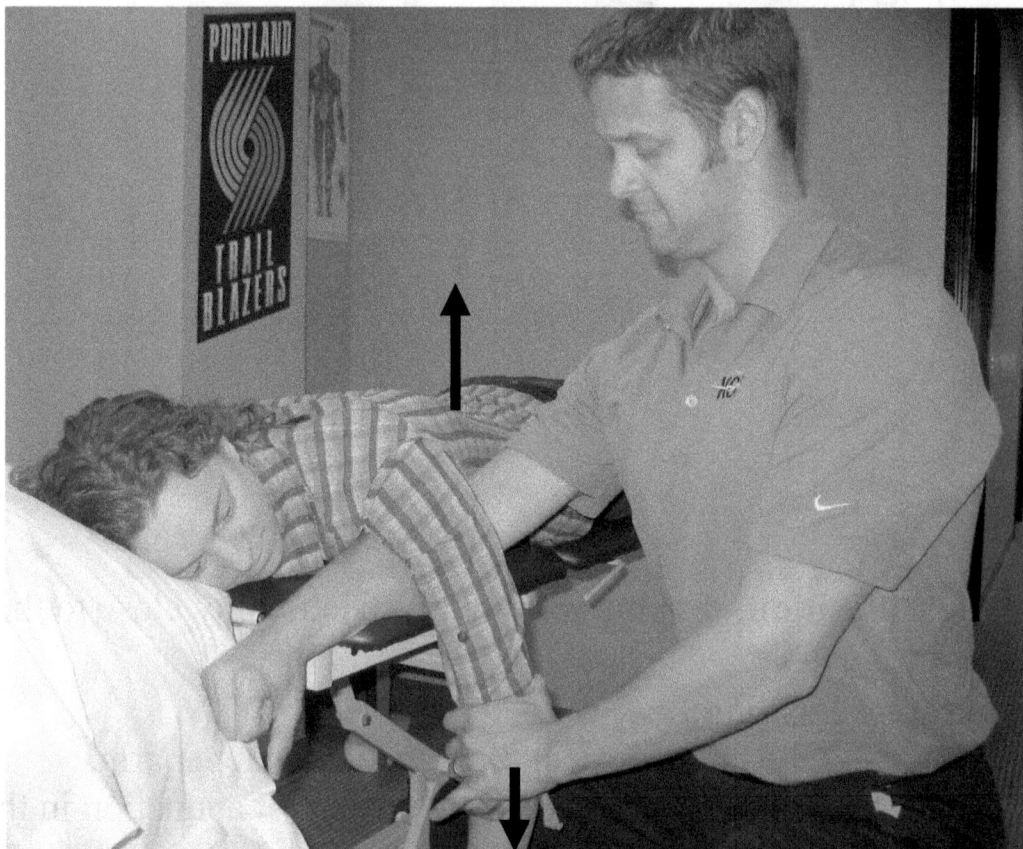

- **Patient Position:** Lying on their stomach.
- **Therapist Position:**
    - Facing the patient's upper arm.
    - The therapist puts their closest forearm under the anterior part of the glenohumeral joint.
    - The therapist's other hand is placed just proximal to the elbow.
    - While pushing up on the patient's glenohumeral joint with their forearm, the therapist also pulls down on the elbow to create a stretch on the posterior aspect of the glenohumeral joint.
    - Mobilize 10-15 times, reset, and repeat 2-3 times.

Exercises and Patient Self Mobilizations

Exercise guidelines:

- 2-3 intensity sessions per week 20-50 min
- 3-5 sets of 2-3 exercises specific to the muscles that need strengthening
- 3-6 reps most effective for increasing max dynamic strength
- 6-12 reps target muscle hypertrophy/ best combination of load and volume
- 12-15 reps rarely increases max strength – muscle endurance
- Various loading strategies = optimal strength, hypertrophy and muscle endurance
- To maintain strength, lift 1-2 times per week

Kramer & Ratamess *Fundamentals of resistance training: Progression and Ex prescription Med Sci Sports & Ex 2004*

Beginning Exercises

One Arm Row

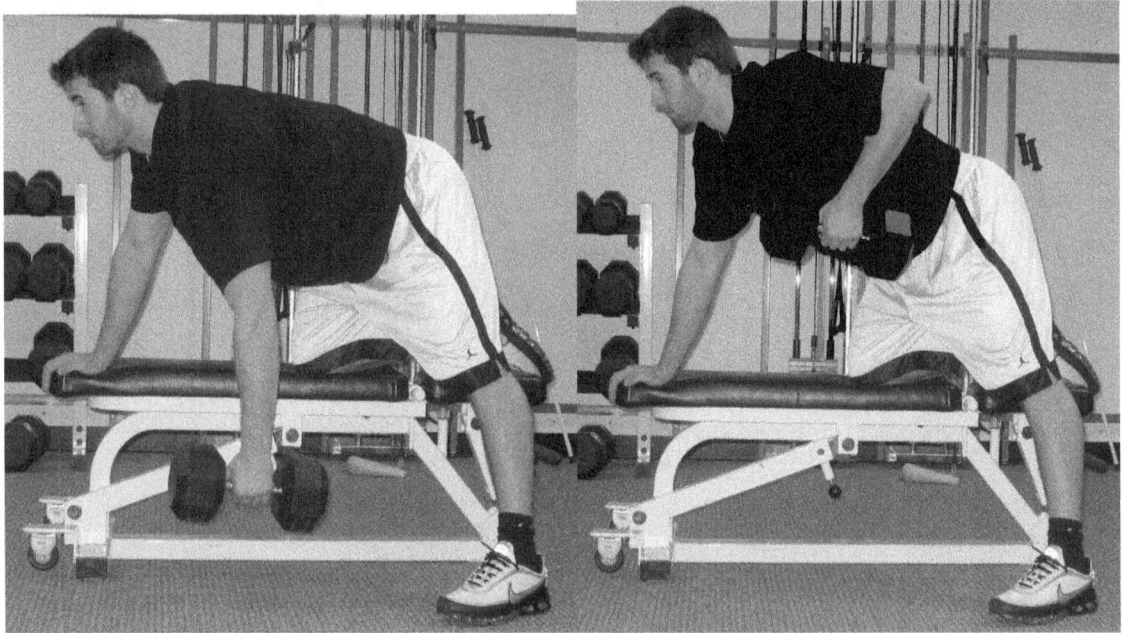

- This exercise is best performed on a bench as shown above.
- Make sure that you form a stable base with the non-working arm and the leg on that same side. Keep the back flat as shown above, and do not hunch over the weight.
- As you lift the weight up, squeeze the shoulder blade towards the middle of your back.
- When lowering the weight make sure that it is under control and do not just let it fall down.

Bench and Reach

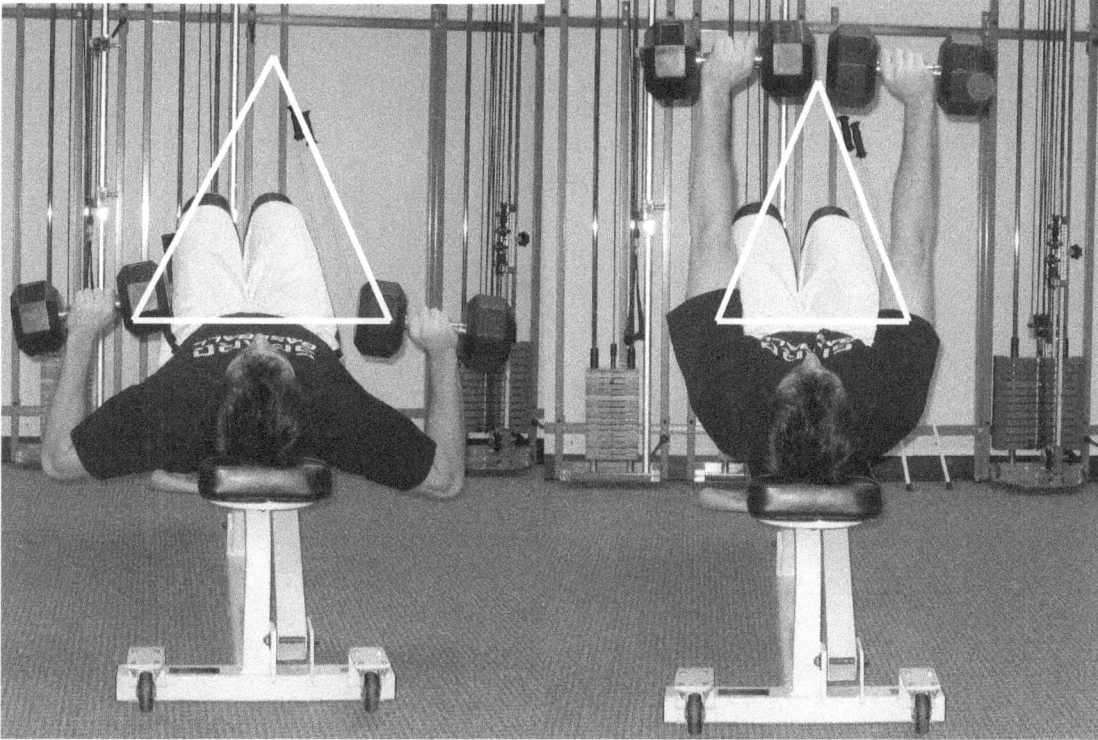

- There has been some controversy as to whether a baseball player should do an exercise like this, but this exercise is very important to the development of the serratus anterior muscle.
- This particular muscle is one of the most important muscles in a baseball athlete, especially the pitcher.
- This exercise begins with the weight at the shoulders (think of that position as the base of the triangle) and finishes with the weight at the top with the shoulder blades off the bench (the top of the triangle).
- Again, make sure to lower the weight under control.

Scapular Retraction

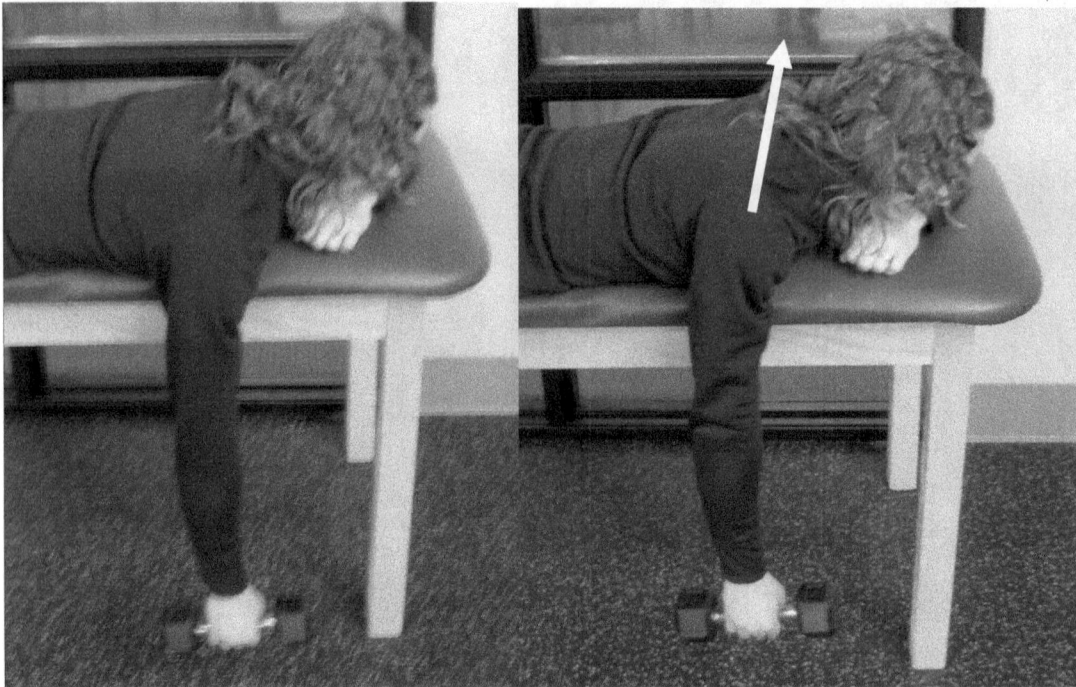

- Lock the elbow straight.
- Move the shoulder blade upwards towards the spine.

Mid Trap Lift

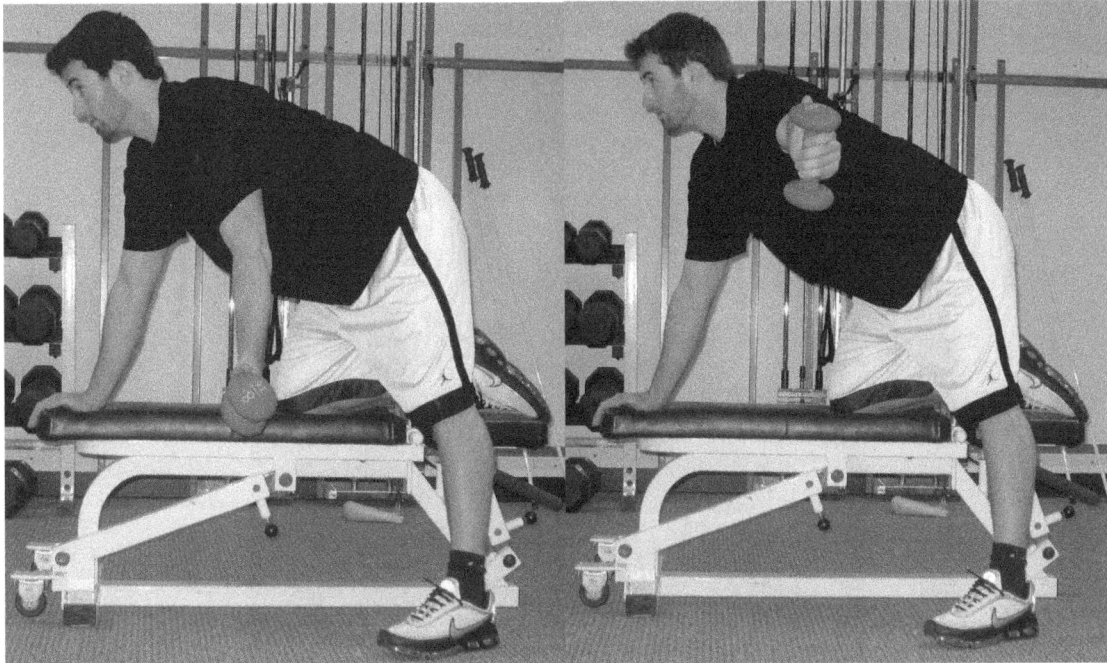

- This exercise works the stabilizer muscles in the back.
- They also help to control the deceleration of the arm.
- Make sure that your thumb is turned up as shown in the picture, and that you are squeezing your shoulder blade towards your backbone as you lift the weight.

Lower Trap Lift (45 degrees)

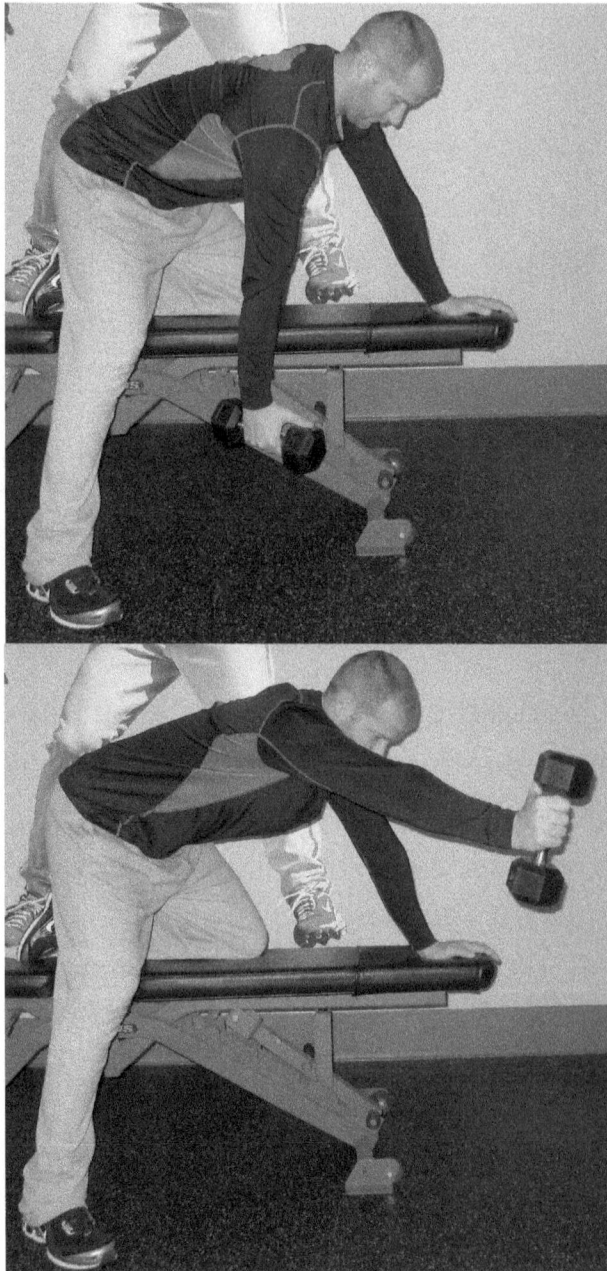

- Place arm in a thumbs-up position.
- Lift upwards maintaining a 145° angle between arm and body or 45° angle to the floor.

Shoulder External Rotation with Pulley
(Infraspinatus)

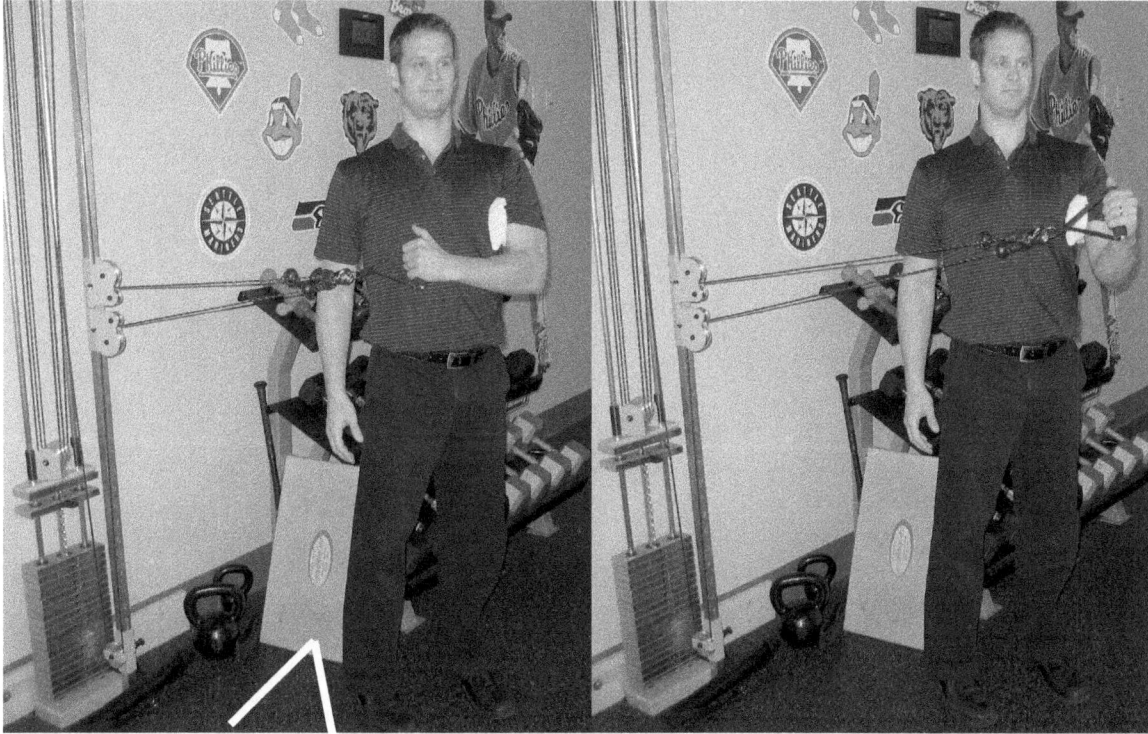

- Stand with feet at a 45 degree angle to the pulley
- With a towel under the involved arm, rotate the arm out so that it is neutral with the body.

Shoulder External Rotation on Bent Knee

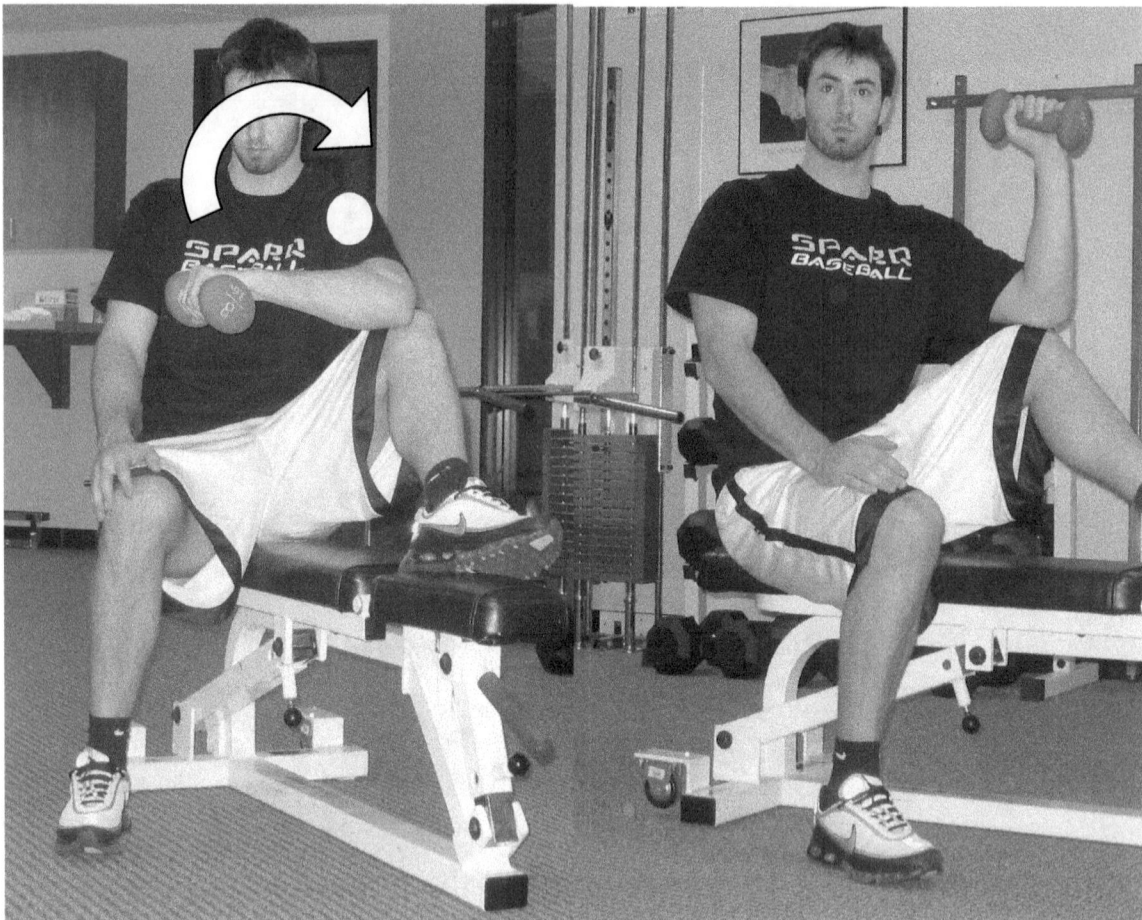

- This exercise works both the infraspinatus and supraspinatus
- Start off with the weight at knee height and rotate your arm up towards the ceiling
- Make sure that the elbow does not straighten and that the shoulder stays down and does not rock.

Subscap Lift

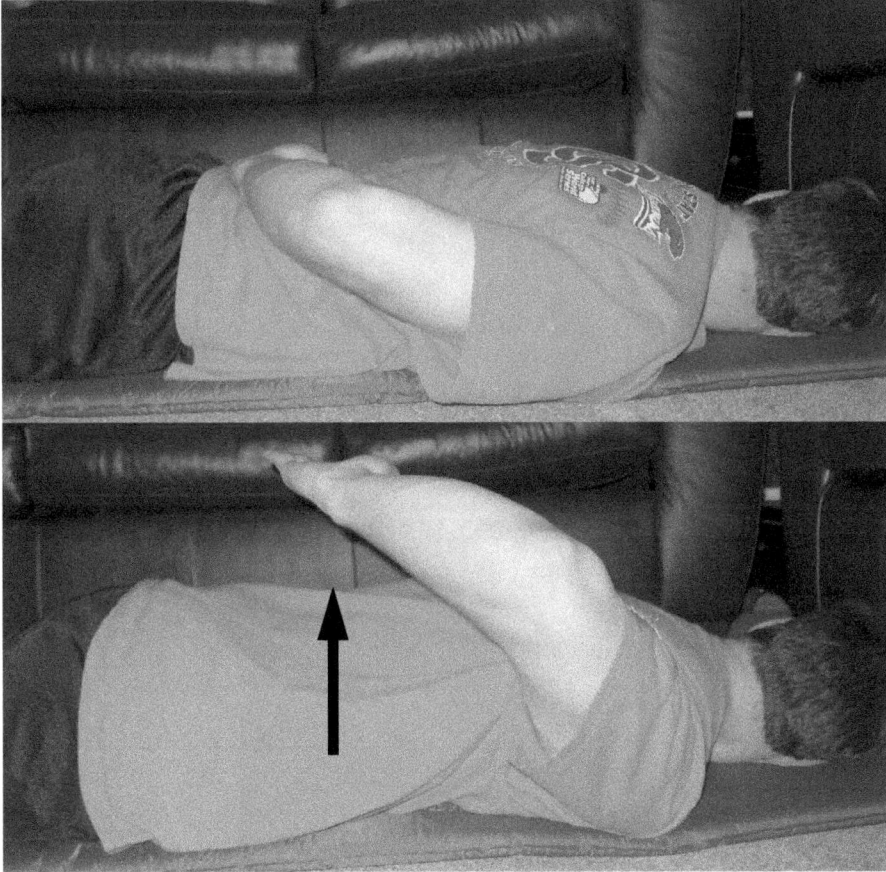

- Lay on your stomach with your pitching arm on top of your back.
- While keeping the elbow bent, lift your entire arm up towards the ceiling.
- Start with no weight on this one…it is a hard exercise.

Standing Biceps Curls

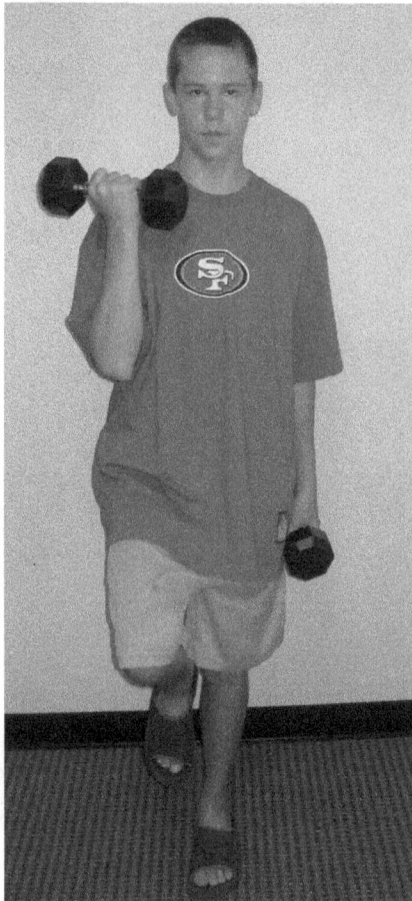

- Start with 2 dumbbells in each hand, with palms facing in.
- Lift one arm up, towards your shoulder, bending at the elbow.
- While lifting the weight also turn your hand so that the palm ends up facing your shoulder at the top.
- For added difficultly, stand on one leg

Triceps Extension

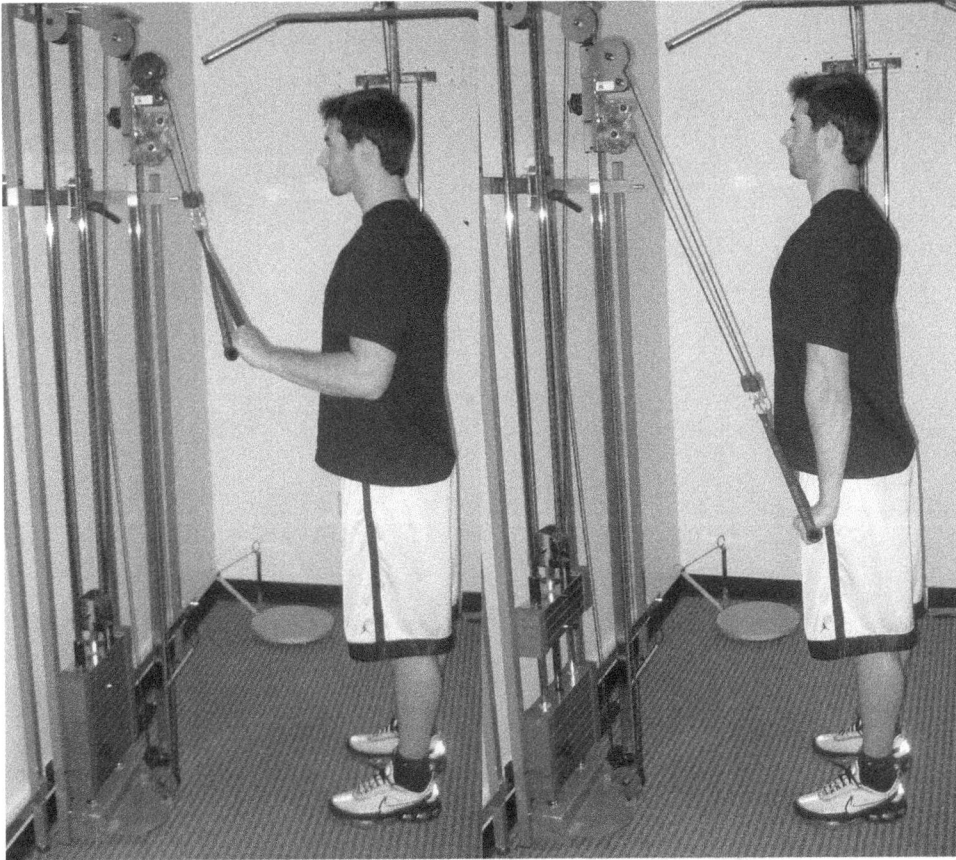

- This exercise works to strengthen the back of the arm and to help protect the elbow along with the biceps curls.
- We prefer this exercise because it really isolates the triceps without putting additional stress on the shoulder like some other triceps exercises do.
- It is important to keep your elbow close to your trunk when doing this exercise so that you are not cheating and using other muscles.

Intermediate Exercises
Dynamic Hug

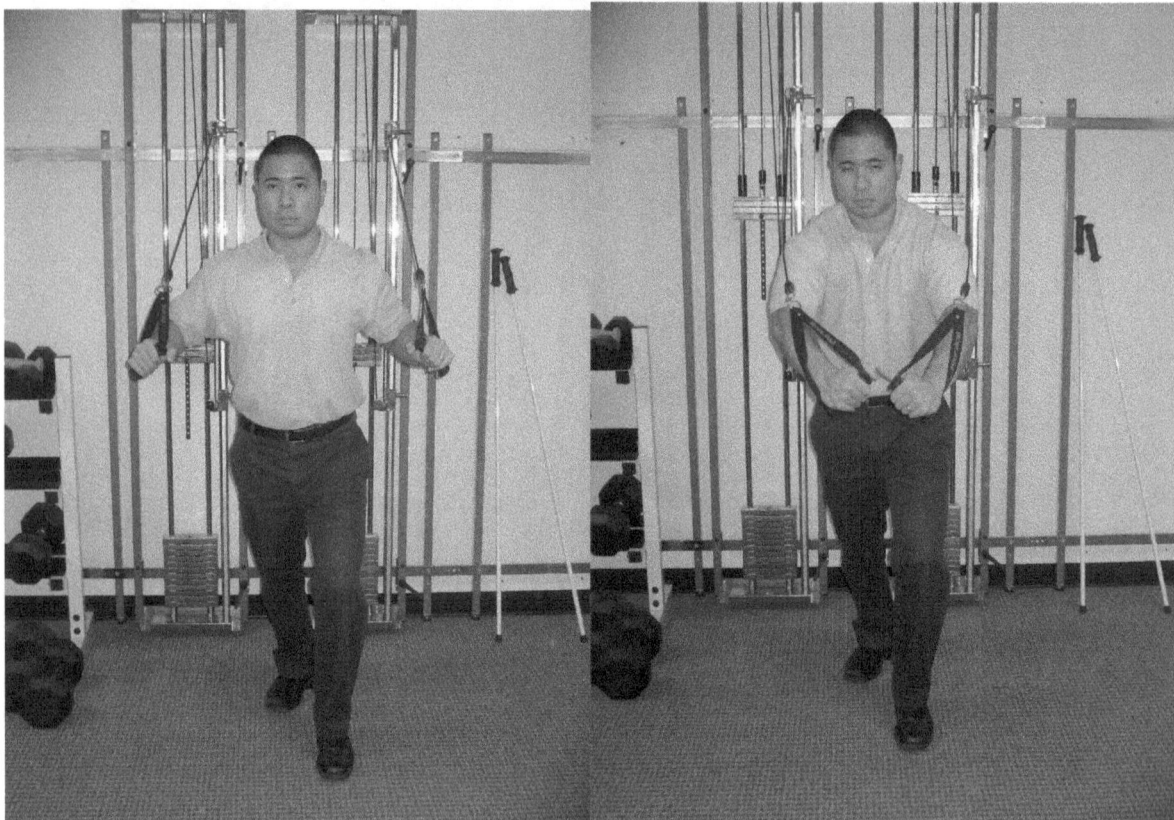

- Face away from the pulleys which should be spaced slightly wider than shoulder width
- Keep your arms slightly lower than your shoulder (60 deg elevation)
- Press forward, like you are hugging a tree
- Return to the starting position under control

Lat pulldown

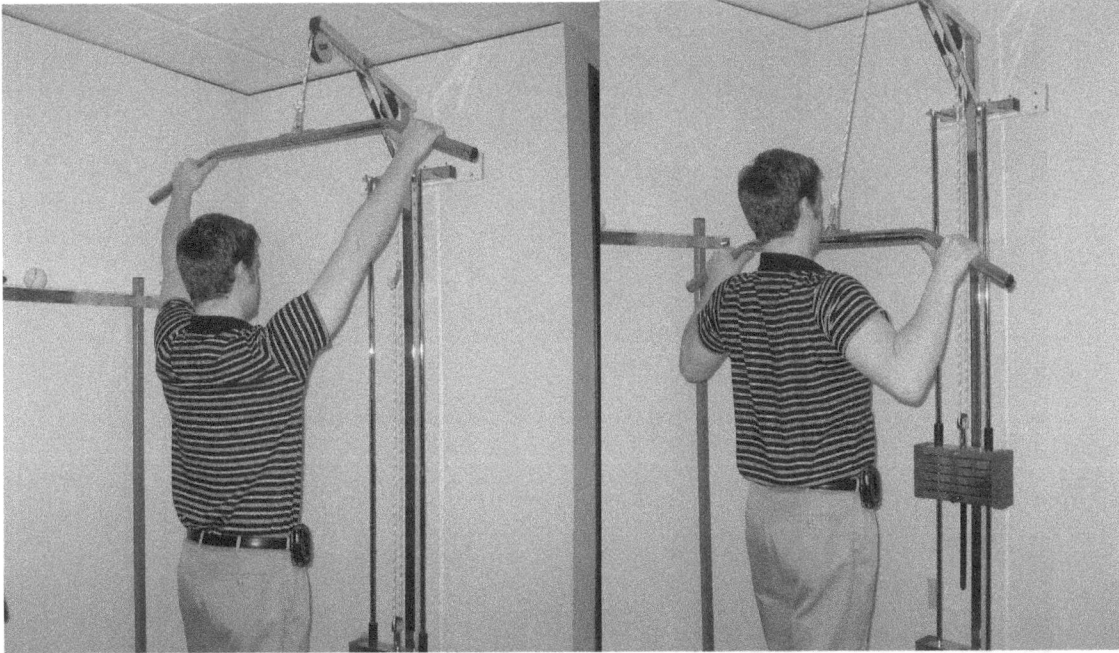

- Place your hands a little further out than shoulder width
- Lean back slightly
- Pull the bar down to your chest (never to the back of your neck)
- Control the bar back to its return position

Shoulder Lift on Table

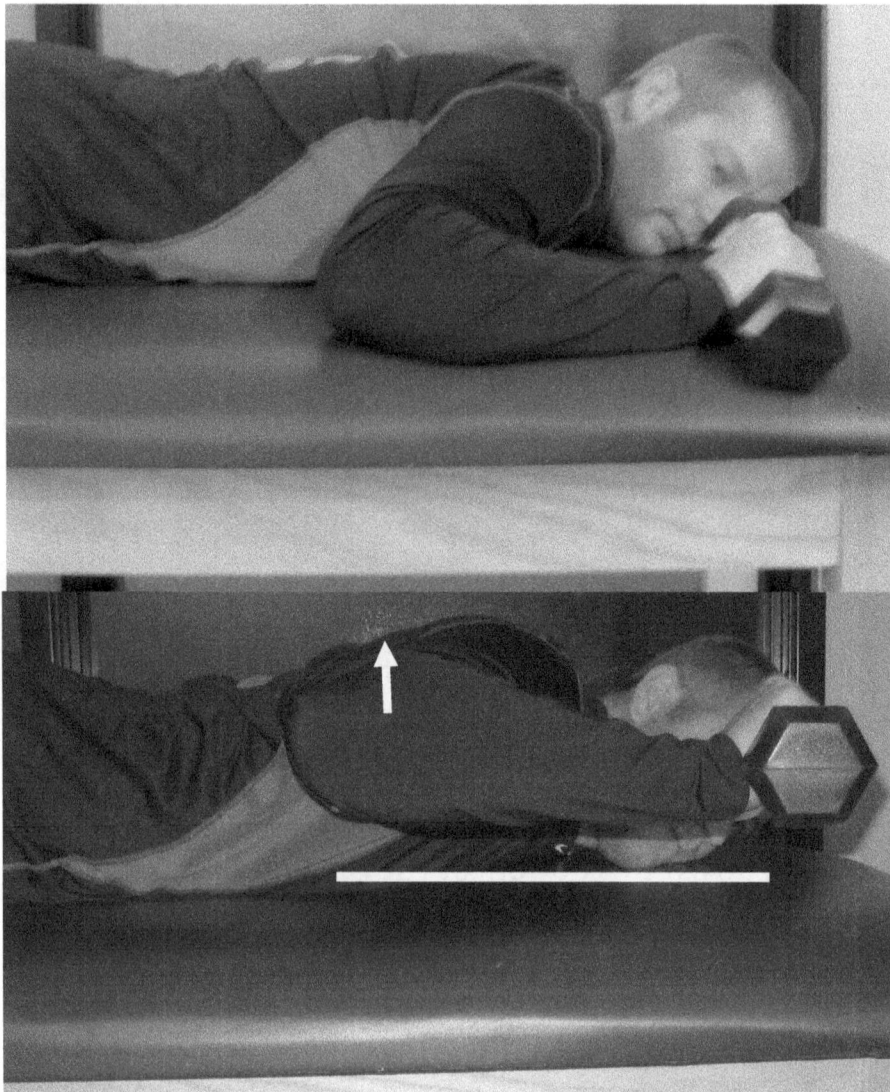

- Bend at the elbow and maintain this 90°/90° position of shoulder/elbow
- Lift the shoulder, elbow, and wrist off the table and return to the starting position slowly (count of 3-5 secs).
- Try to keep the forearm level to the table.

Full Shoulder Rotation Lift

1

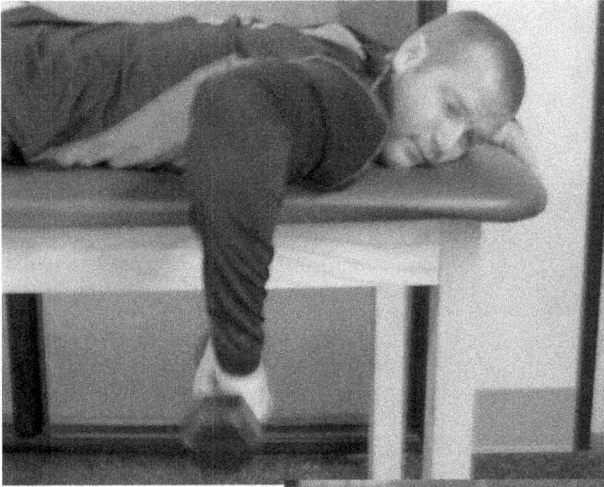

2

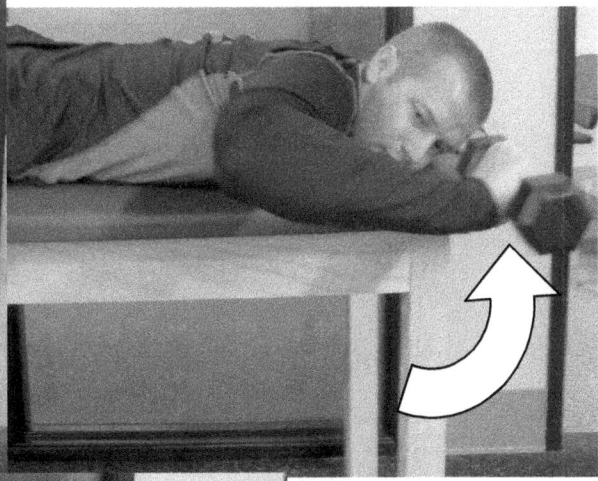

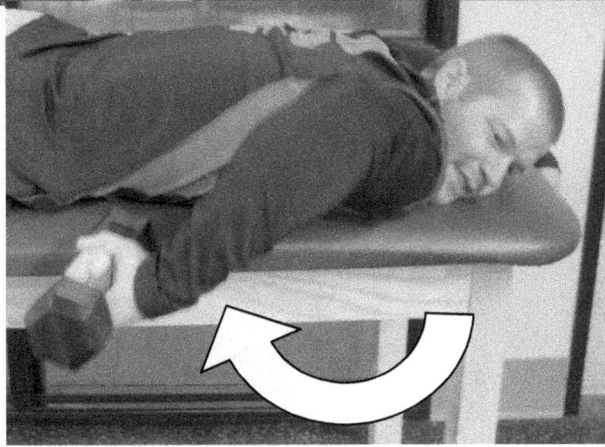

3

- Start off lying on the stomach and having the weight below with the elbow bent as seen in picture 1.
- First rotate the arm up towards the head as seen in picture 2.
- Then rotate the weight back towards the hip as seen in picture 3.
- This exercise needs to be performed slowly (3-5 secs) each direction.

90/90 Shoulder External Rotation with Pulley

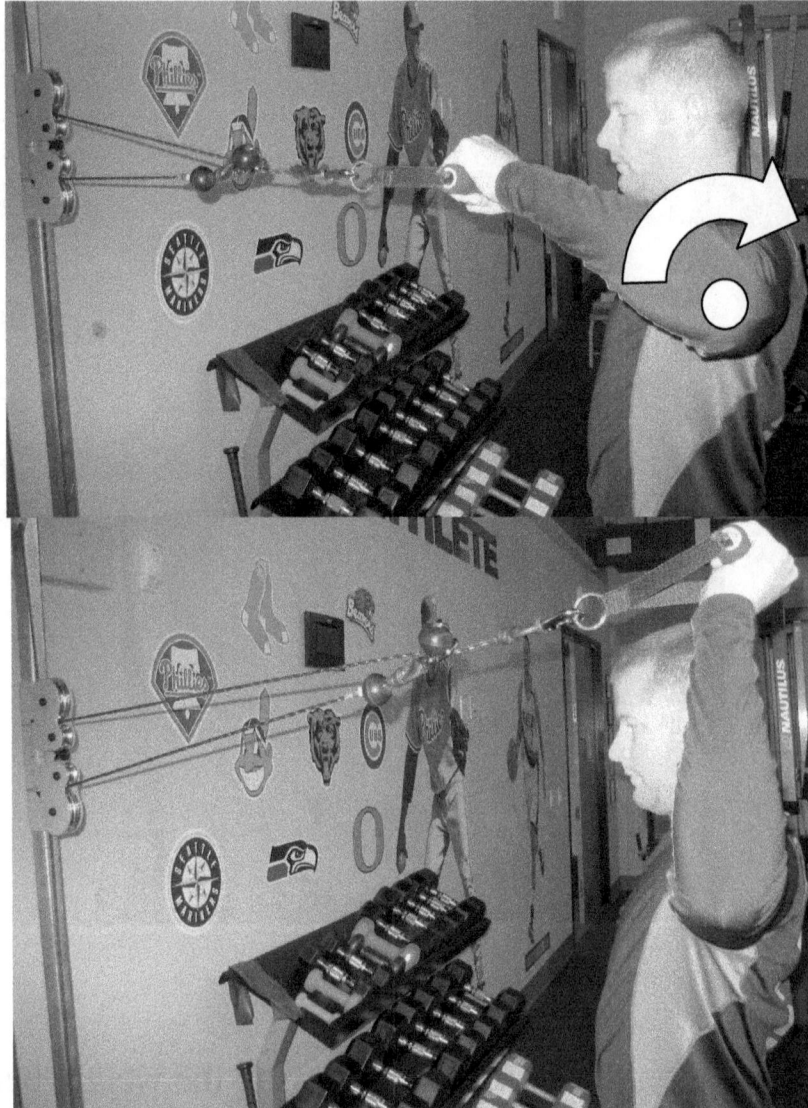

- Stand facing the pulley, with the pulley slightly below the shoulder
- While keeping the elbow bent, rotate the arm backwards
- Keep the shoulder joint still and do not rock the joint to move the weight

Pulley Bicep Curl

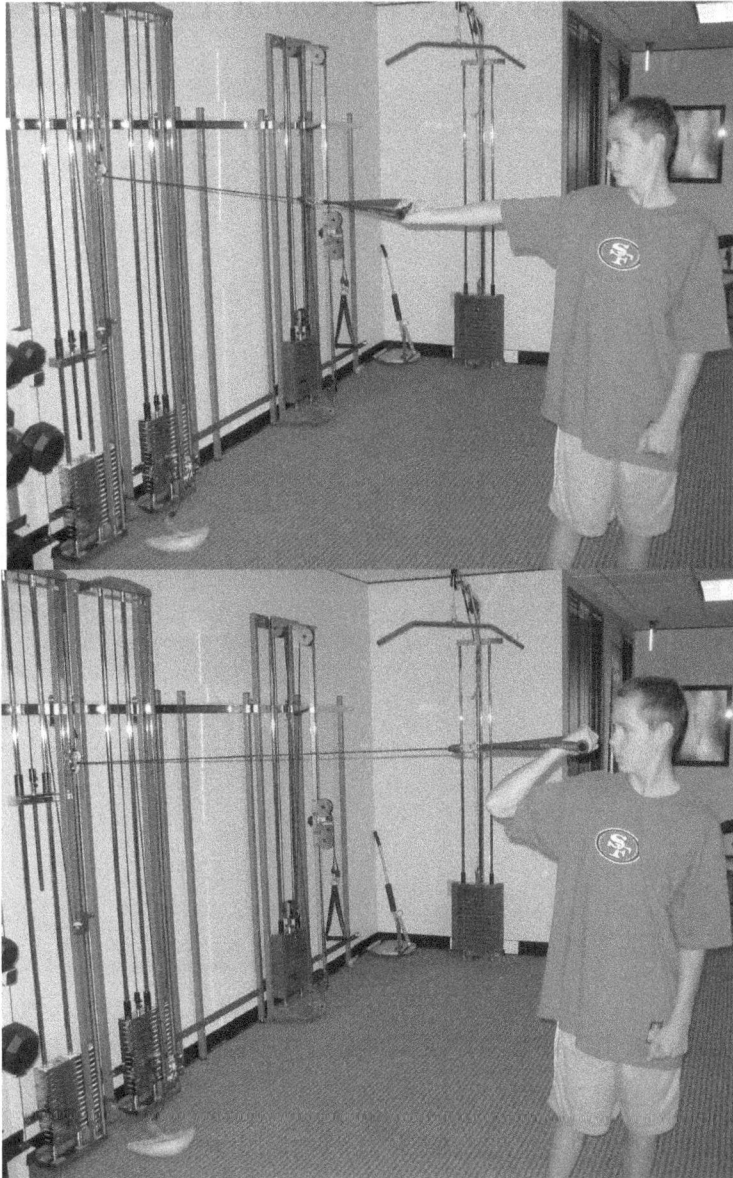

- Stand with the pulley height slightly above the shoulder
- Bend the elbow while making sure that the hand does not travel forward
- Slowly lower the weight back to the starting position

Advanced Shoulder Exercises
Serratus Anterior Lift

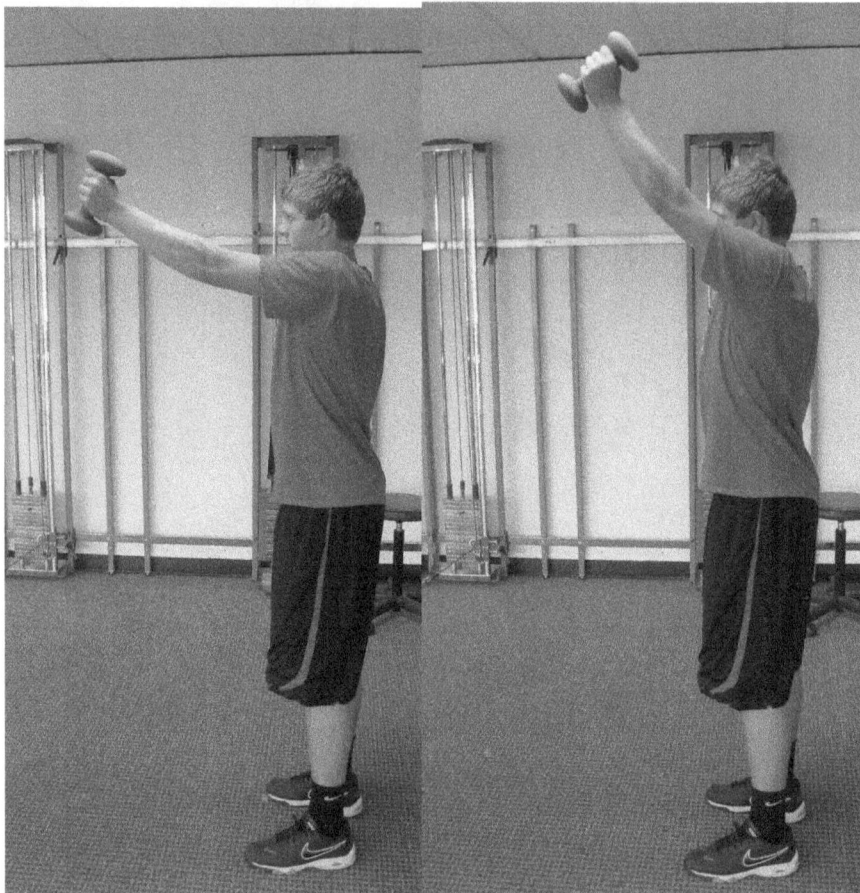

- While standing, hold a weight out in front of you as shown, slightly above parallel.
- Keeping the thumb up, raise the weight up, above your head.
- Lower the weight to starting position and repeat.

Ball Push Up

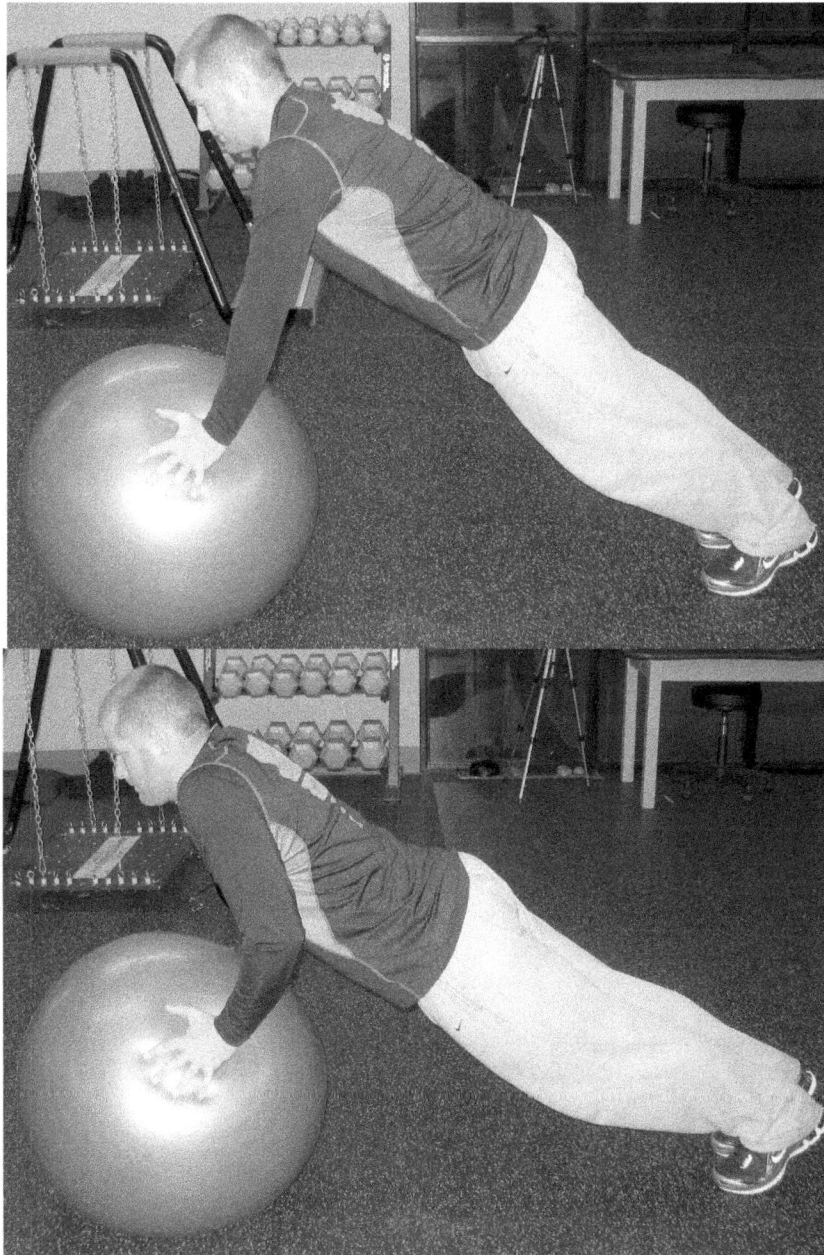

- Start by placing the hands on the ball, a little more than shoulder width apart, and your feet slightly more than hip width apart.
- Keeping the back straight, lower the body towards the ball and then press up.

Internal Rotation Toss

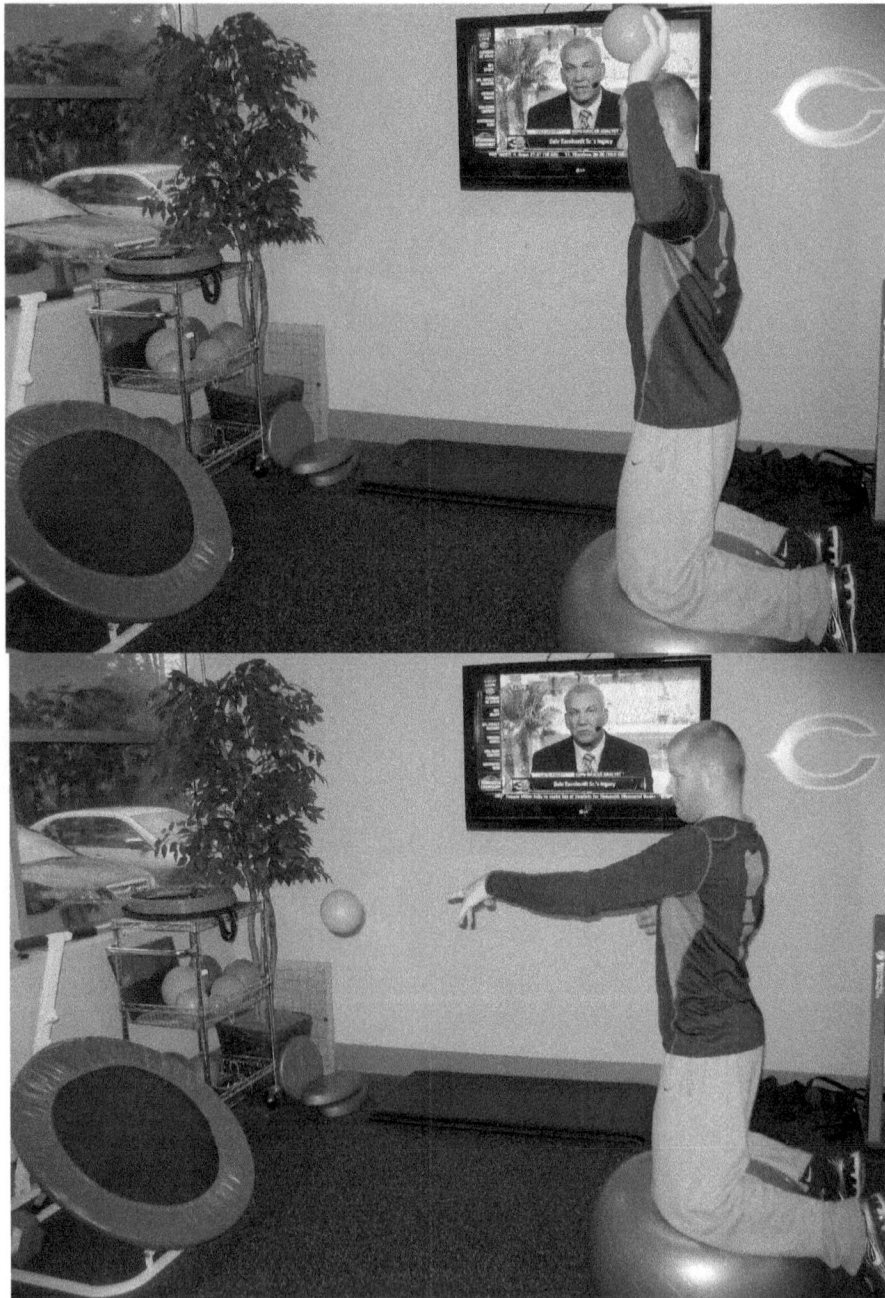

- Start with the arm in the 90/90 position and kneeling on a ball. If not able to kneel on a ball then kneel on the ground.
- Throw the ball into a rebounder / trampoline and catch and absorb the force and immediately toss again.

Cross Body Shoulder Lift

1

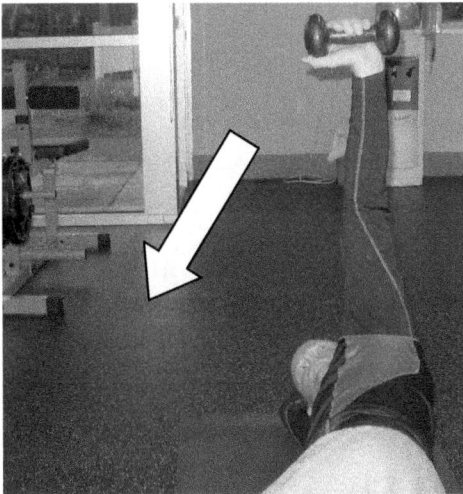

2

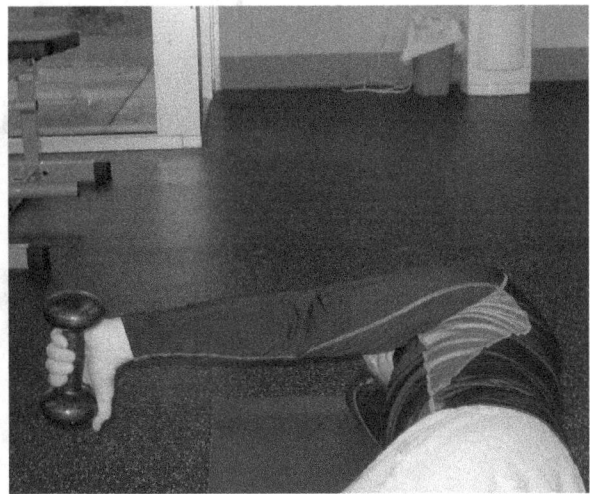

3

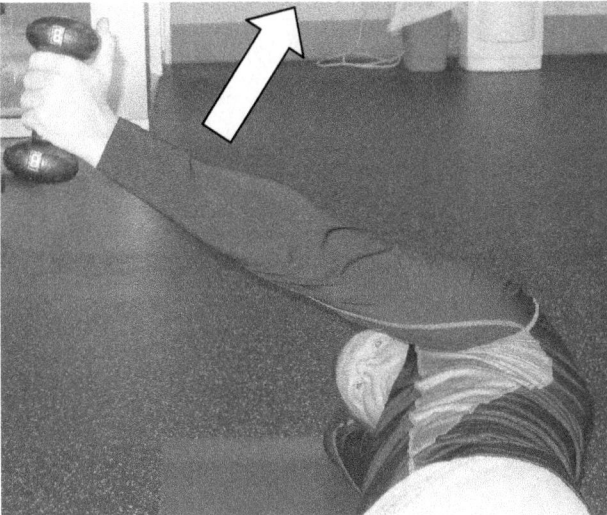

4

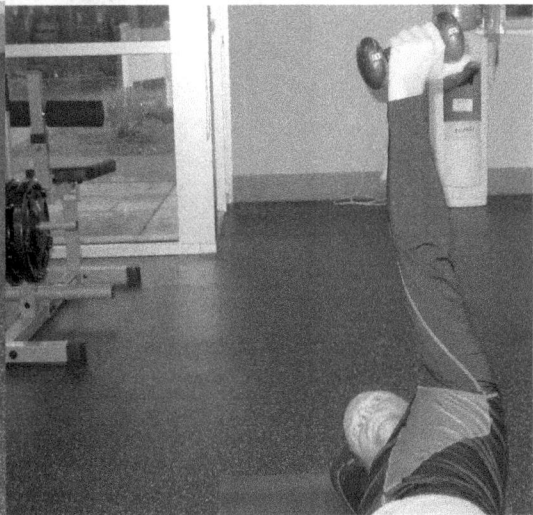

- Start with the elbow locked overhead and the thumb pointed down (Pic 1).
- Slowly lower the weight down to the floor (Pic 2).
- Just before the thumb / weight touches the floor, rotate the thumb up towards the ceiling (Pic 3) and return to the starting position (Pic 4).

Internal Rotation with Pulley

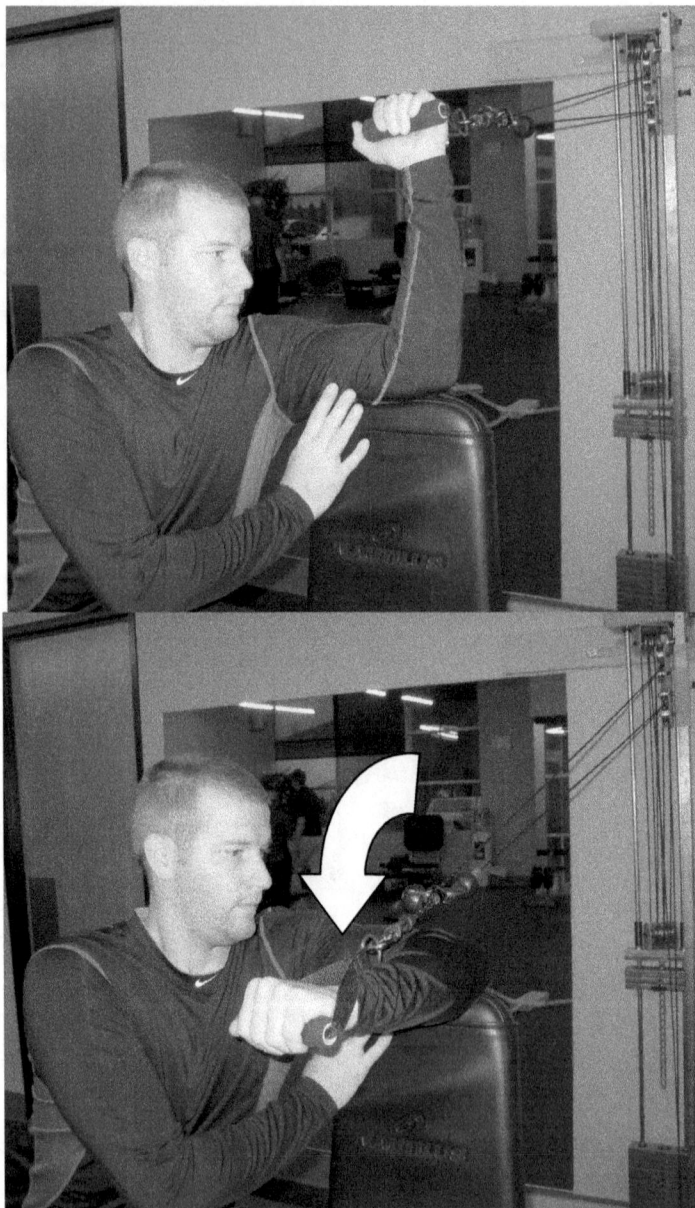

- Grab a pulley that is above shoulder height while in standing and place an elbow on a bench
- Rotate the hand down so that the forearm is parallel with the ground
- Slowly return to the starting position and repeat

Self Stretches

Prone Internal Rotation Hang

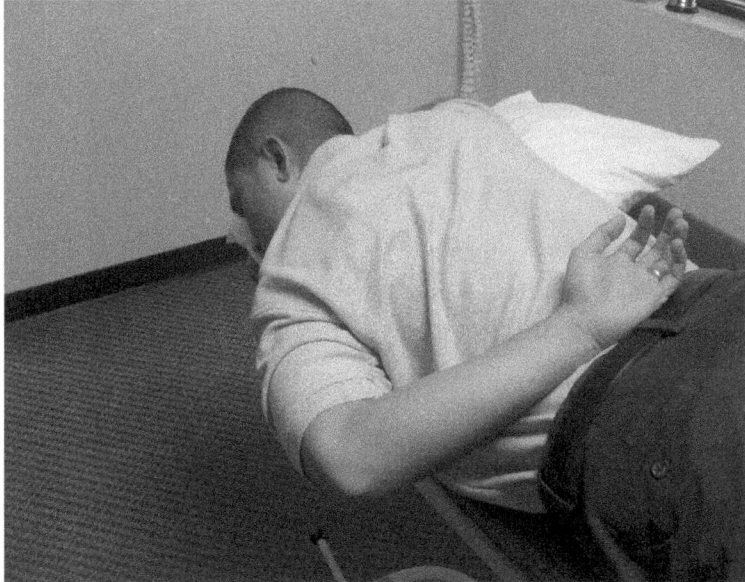

- **Patient Position:** Lie on stomach with involved arm on your back.
- Let your elbow drop to floor.
- Hold for 2-3 minutes, reset and repeat 2-3 times.

Izumi T, Aoki M, et al: Stretching positions for the posterior capsule of the glenohumeral joint. Amer J Sports Med 36: 2014-2022.

Sleeper Stretch

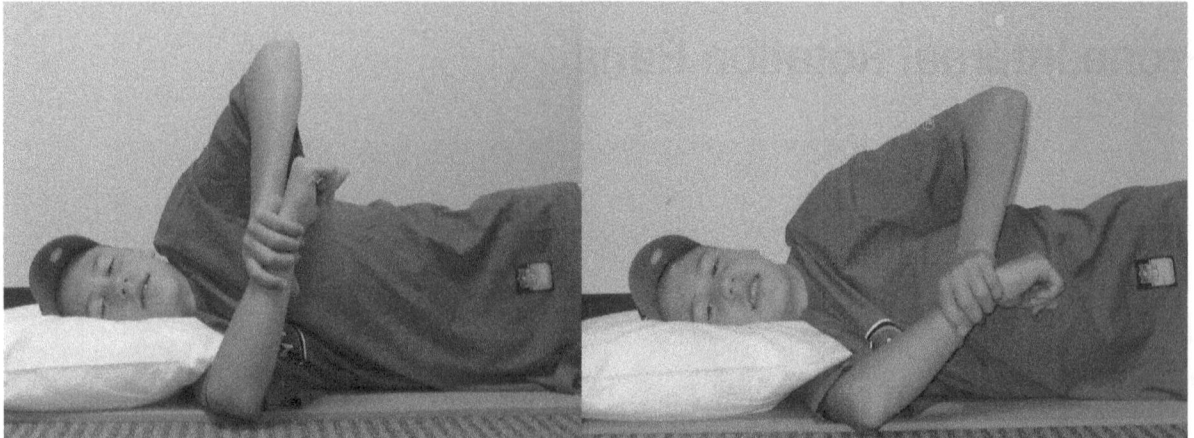

- This stretch needs to be performed at least 3 times for 30 seconds up to 3 minutes
- Make sure that you do not push so hard that your shoulder comes up and touches your chin.
- You should feel a slight discomfort in the back of your shoulder, NOT the front. If you feel a discomfort in the front of your shoulder, talk to your therapist.

Cooper J in Donatelli RA, *Physical Therapy of the Shoulder*. 4th Ed. 2004, Missouri: Elsevier.

About the Authors:

Donn Dimond, PT, OCS
Physical Therapist, Board Certified in Orthopedic Physical Therapy

Donn currently owns The KOR Physical Therapy in Portland, OR. His practice encompasses many levels of patients from high level athletes to the general population. Donn has worked with many athletes, from little leagues to the Professional level. Donn is a contributing author to Dr. Donatelli's *Sports Specific Rehabilitation, Orthopedic Physical Therapy*, and *Physical Therapy of the Shoulder 5th ed*. Donn lectures nationally to other physical therapists on how to assess and treat patients with shoulder injuries along with lecturing on high level performance training for various athletes.

Robert Donatelli, PhD, PT, Orthopedic Certified Specialist
National Director of Sports Specific Rehabilitation and Performance Enhancement Programs, Physiotherapy Associates, Las Vegas, NV

Dr. Donatelli has worked with numerous professional athletes including Marquis Grissom (San Francisco Giants), Michael Barrett (Chicago Cubs), Brian Jordan (Atlanta Braves), Dale Murphy (Atlanta Braves), Tony Armis (Montreal Expos), Terrance Newman (Dallas Cowboys), Matt Stenchcome (Tampa Bay Buccaneers) and many more.

Dr. Donatelli served as a member of the PBATS (Professional Baseball Athletic Trainers Society) Research Committee from 1996-2001. In addition, he has served as a physical therapy consultant to the Montreal Expos, Philadelphia Phillies, and Milwaukee Brewers baseball teams.

Dr. Donatelli has published four textbooks – Physical Therapy of the Shoulder 4th Ed, Orthopedic Physical Therapy 3rd Ed, Biomechanics of the Foot and Ankle 2nd Ed, and Sports Specific Rehabilitation, 2006. Dr. Donatelli has published over 25 articles in peer review journals. Dr. Donatelli lectures throughout the United States, Canada, England, Ireland, Scotland, Australia, Iceland, and lectured at the Swedish Foot and Ankle Society. In addition, Dr. Donatelli was the keynote speaker for the Romanian Physical Therapy Association from 2003 thru 2008.

Kent Morimatsu, DPT
Physical Therapist

Kent is currently a therapist who specializes in treating overhead athletes in Portland, OR. Kent has worked with numerous athletes from high school to the pros.

<u>Notes</u>

_____

_____

_____

_____

_____

_____

_____

_____

_____

_____

_____

_____

_____

_____

_____

_____

_____

_____

_____

_____

_____

www.ingramcontent.com/pod-product-compliance
Lightning Source LLC
Chambersburg PA
CBHW061821210326
41599CB00034B/7074